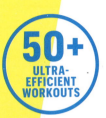

50+
ULTRA-
EFFICIENT
WORKOUTS

Men'sHealth

7-MINUTE WORKOUTS

FOR FAT BURN

BY **ANDREW HEFFERNAN, CSCS**
AND THE EDITORS OF MEN'S HEALTH

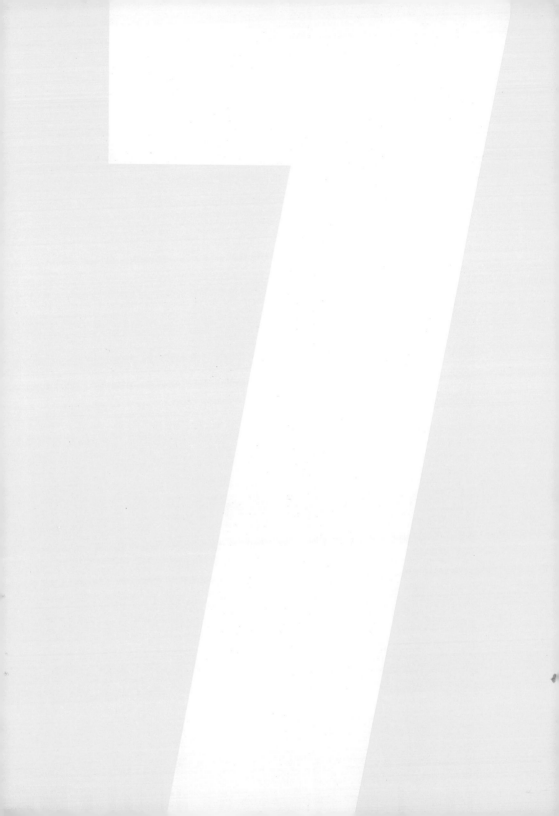

INTRODUCTION

YOUR FITNESS JOURNEY doesn't start with a leap, a jump, or a TikTok-worthy backflip. All you need to do is take the tiniest of steps. And that step only needs to last a few minutes.

We get it. Working out can feel intimidating. Life experience, social media, and your last visit to Orangetheory have taught you that every workout should be an hour-long sweatfest, leaving you broken, barely able to crawl home. And fitness mags and websites have deluged you with dynamic warm-ups and cooldowns and drop sets, plus a host of other terms that make little sense. So where do you even begin?

Answer: Start with seven minutes. Because the key to any fitness goal, from losing weight to building muscle to mastering that backflip, is getting started—and it's hard to get started in fitness when you're paralyzed by fear and frustration.

The seven-minute workout is the antidote for that paralysis—and we've collected more than 50 of them in this guide. No, it's not easy to commit 30 minutes or 60 minutes or 120 minutes to fitness every day. But just about everyone can find seven minutes in their schedule, whether that means leaving happy hour seven minutes early, going to bed seven minutes late, or banging out pushups during the first seven minutes of a Netflix marathon. And that means you can commit to seven minutes of potentially life-changing fitness.

No, seven minutes a day won't transform you into Marvel's newest Captain America, but it will help you crush calories and build critical muscle. By taking on exactly one manageable, bite-sized session, you'll be showing up for your body and your fitness every single day, and that will spark more change in your body than you realize. Seven minutes is enough time to kick-start better bloodflow throughout your body, and it's enough time to push your heart rate into the stratosphere. And according to one 2013 study in the American College of Sports Medicine's Health and Fitness Journal, seven minutes is enough to improve strength and endurance while also burning fat.

Perhaps more important than all that: It's enough time to build a fitness habit. Every day you train for seven minutes, you're carving out time for your health and just a little bit of sweat. Soon enough, your mind realizes you can take more, and seven minutes leads to seven ultra-intense minutes—and that leads to 14 minutes a day. And 21. And . . . you get the point.

I've seen it work. I frequently start time-strapped clients with daily seven-minute workouts. Eventually, they almost always want more. One recent client went from simple seven-minute workouts to lengthier sessions that included everything from deadlifts to step-ups to sprint sessions on her Concept2 rower. Another client dropped 25 pounds.

It all starts with seven minutes of training. Commit to that now, and the results will follow.

EBENEZER SAMUEL, CSCS
FITNESS DIRECTOR
MEN'S HEALTH

TABLE OF CONTENTS

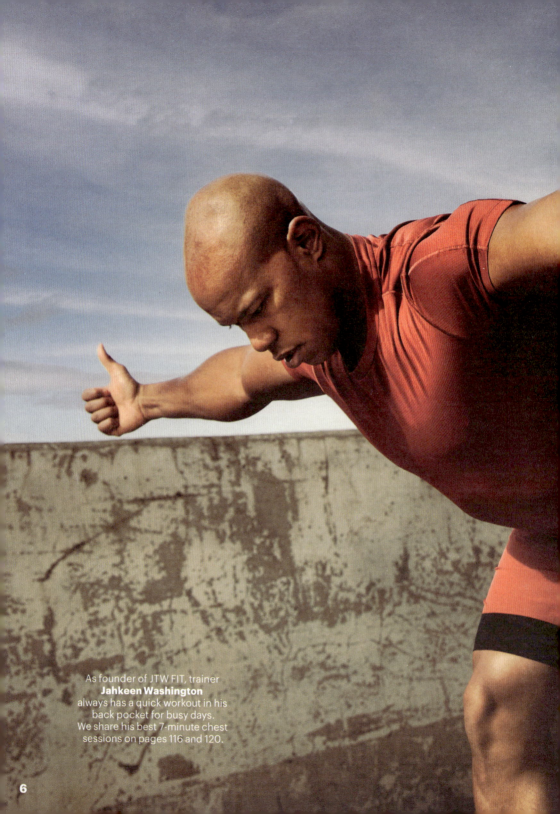

As founder of JTW FIT, trainer **Jahkeen Washington** always has a quick workout in his back pocket for busy days. We share his best 7-minute chest sessions on pages 116 and 120.

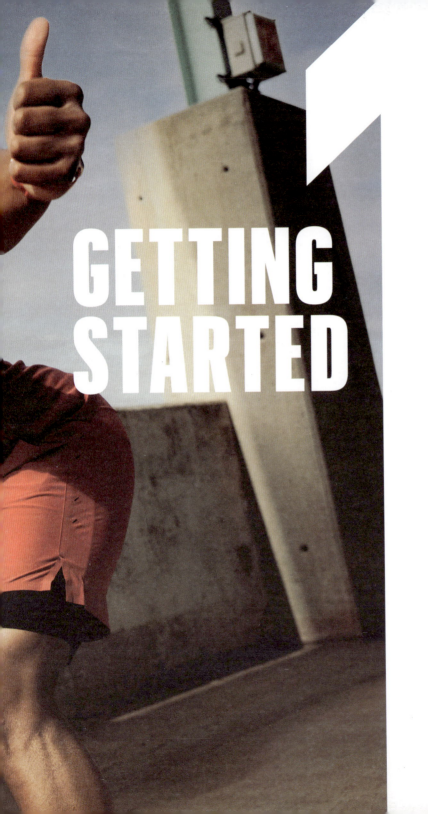

GETTING STARTED

1

WHY SEVEN MINUTES IS ALL YOU NEED

WE LIVE IN A MORE-IS-BETTER WORLD.

Most of us believe that if a little of something is effective, then a lot of it must be more so. Working longer, playing harder, and going the extra mile—it's all part of the get-ahead treadmill.

A lot of us take the same approach to exercise: If three workouts a week are good, six must be even better. If one set of each movement is good, four must be your ticket to superhero status. And come hell or high water, we're going to get those workouts in.

But when it comes to your body, "more is better" can be a big mistake.

Sure, there's a time and a place for long, involved workouts. When you have the time and energy and space to eat, sleep, and recover properly, spending an hour or more in the gym a few times a week can net you some decent fitness gains.

But what about when you're drowning in stress? When you barely have a minute to yourself? When the gym sounds as appealing as Grand Central at rush hour?

That's exactly the wrong time to triple down on your workouts, and the right time to turn to the workouts in this book: They'll challenge you, keep you strong, keep fat at bay, and build muscle—all with the barest minimum time commitment from you.

There are tons of other books and articles and trainers who will show you what to do when you have plenty of time and space for exercise. This book is for the many times when you have neither.

Beginners will discover an effective but highly doable entry point for exercise that long, involved, equipment-heavy programs can't duplicate. Intermediates will enjoy experimenting with dozens of novel at-home moves and workouts they can use to add to—or replace—their current repertoire. More advanced folks will round out their training knowledge with new workout strategies that they can use as quick-hitting finishers.

And exercisers of all levels will finally have an effective option they can stick to when time is tightest and stress is highest.

A word on that for hardcore folks who insist on sticking to a time-consuming workout program 365 days a year: You may think your body is a machine, capable of recovery regardless of whatever else is going on in your life. You may think that the way to build fitness is to keep piling on the sets and reps, even when you're run-down, achy, and stressed to the gills. You may think you're a superhero.

But trust us on this: Much as you may think you're Iron Man or the Hulk, you actually have more in common with the tree-creature Groot, from *Guardians of the Galaxy*. Made entirely of live wood, Groot is plenty strong, but he's easily wounded. He needs time and patience to recover from shocks and injuries.

That's you, too: When you push the gas on your workouts at the wrong time, with too little recovery and not enough of the right fuel, you end up with zero progress—and you risk injury as well. Exercise is a stressor, and when you pile stress on top of more stress, you're asking for trouble, Mr. Tree Creature. Think you're safe if you don't have

a physical job? Think again: Recent data from the *Journal of Strength and Conditioning Research* shows that psychological stress slows recovery from exercise.

So whether you're just starting on your fitness journey or you're looking for ways to streamline a lifelong discipline—we've got you covered.

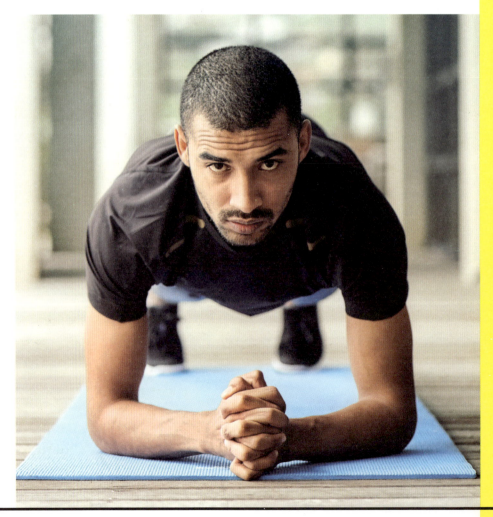

WHAT ARE SEVEN-MINUTE WORKOUTS GOOD FOR?

THE MILLION-DOLLAR QUESTION: Do seven-minute workouts...work? Regardless of your fitness goals, the answer is yes. Let's run through a few of the most common goals out there, and show how this approach can help you accomplish each one.

SEVEN-MINUTE WORKOUTS BUILD STRENGTH AND MUSCLE

Think you can't get strong and build muscle without tons of weights and eons of time? Short workouts have been a staple in the workout programs of some of the strongest and most muscular folks in history.

Consider the case of a Swedish gym owner named Willum.

"Willum was too cheap to hire help," recalls bodybuilding coach Menno Henselmans, ISSA, who worked with the Swede early on. As a result, he was the gym's everything guy: front desk man, floor cleaner, plumber, head trainer. Never had more than a few minutes to himself from morning till night.

But that didn't stop Willum from building an impressive physique.

"Instead of working out all at once, he exercised in five-minute spurts all day long," says Henselmans: a deadlift here, a set of chin-ups there.

Far from holding him back, the piecemeal approach worked wonders: "The guy was massive," says Henselmans. "Bodybuilder huge."

Or consider the case of Mike Mentzer, one of the thickest bodybuilders ever to tread the stage, who did just one or two hard sets per workout for each of his major muscle groups just three times a week. This is a guy who came within spitting distance of dethroning Arnold Schwarzenegger for the top prize in bodybuilding.

Or consider Casey Viator, a contemporary of Schwarzenegger and Mentzer, who won the Mr. America contest at just 19. He spent much of his career training the same way.

There's more to getting massive than working out,

of course, and in the case of champion bodybuilders, a lot more. But recent science suggests that these three guys—genetic anomalies, to be sure—may well have been onto something.

In 2013, a research study in Scotland compared the strength gains achieved by two sets of male, weight-trained athletes who did upper-body strength exercises three times per week: One group performed three sets of six reps of each move, the other did just one set of six. Eight weeks later, strength gains between the two groups were comparable—with a slight edge to the one-set group.

That's right: The one-set group actually got stronger than the three-set group.

Later that same year, after extensive experimentation with HICT (high-intensity circuit training, an acronym for the seven-minute approach), researchers at the American College of Sports Medicine enumerated how this method could cause improvements in health markers, muscle strength and endurance, and body fat percentage.

In 2019, muscle researcher Dr. Brad Schoenfeld conducted a similar experiment. Three groups

of resistance-trained men performed three full-body strength-training routines three times a week. One group performed one set per exercise; another did three sets, and the final group did five sets.

After eight weeks, the three- and five-set groups built more muscle than the one-set lifters—but that's not the whole story. The one-set group gained strength and endurance comparable to the higher-set groups while also building muscle.

Their workout duration was 13 minutes—about one-third of the time spent by the three-set group.

And those workouts weren't even designed with time efficiency in mind: Had they pushed the tempo on their workouts, they likely could have finished even faster. The workouts in this

book aren't just short versions of regular workouts—they're expertly compressed, so every second of each seven-minute workout is productive: There are no extended rest periods and you don't need to hunt down weights or watch ESPN or amble over to the water fountain or wonder if the guy in the corner is actually going to bench the weight he's got on the bar.

So you're losing less than you think. Strip away nonessentials like those from the average workout, leaving behind only the sets and reps and exercises that will really make a difference in your fitness, and very often, you'll be left with a session lasting not much more than seven minutes.

Two of the smartest and most influential strength coaches of the last 40 years or so—Dan John and Pavel

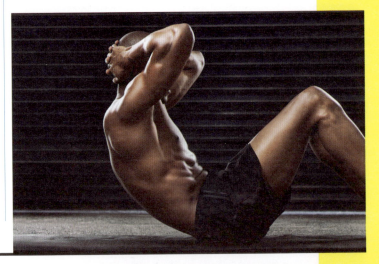

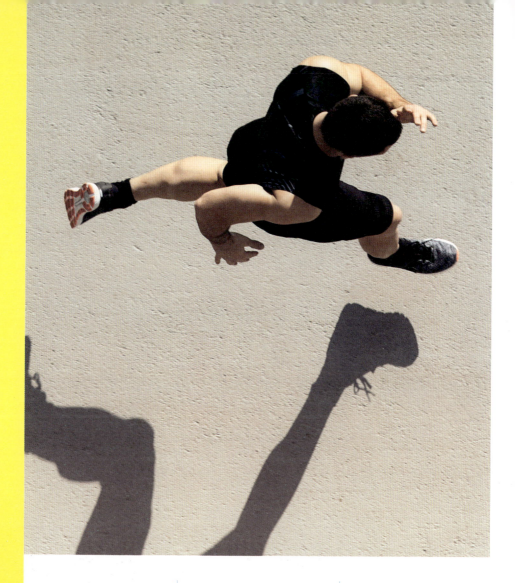

Tsatsouline—both tout workout programs lasting 15 minutes or less per session as among the fastest and safest ways to build strength. For maximum muscle growth—regardless of the constraints of your schedule—Tsatsouline recommends an approach very similar to gym-owner Willum's: short spurts of high effort followed by rest periods that can last as long as several hours.

Can advanced trainees—those looking to reach the very pinnacle of what their bodies can achieve—benefit from more training? In all likelihood, yes—hence the training programs of NFL athletes and military elites. But very few of us are at that level. Most of us just want to look good, avoid injury, and feel energetic and strong as we work and play our way through life. For us, shorter workouts can perform wonders.

SEVEN-MINUTE WORKOUTS
HELP YOU LOSE FAT

Confession: We don't like the phrase *weight loss*. If all you care about is the number on the scale, you can change that by deliberately dehydrating yourself. Fighters do that all the time, and they'll often lose 10 pounds or more by sweating heavily and skipping food and drink for a couple of days. The weight flies off, but they can barely stand, and after five seconds on the scale, they stagger into Popeyes for a 2,000-calorie refeed.

Not exactly a practical or sustainable approach.

What we're really after, then, is *fat loss,* or, more precisely, *body recomposition*—that is, losing fat while retaining, or even gaining, muscle mass. Do that properly and you'll look better, feel better, and perform better—regardless of what happens to your scale weight.

There are three components to successful fat loss. All smart trainers use some version of these, but we're cribbing this specific list from Alwyn Cosgrove,

MS, CSCS—one of the most successful fat-loss trainers in the business.

FAT LOSS REQUIRES:

1. A caloric deficit (eating fewer calories than you burn)

2. Adequate protein consumption

3. A workout program designed to preserve—or build—muscle mass

---

We cover numbers one and two in the nutrition section in this book. They're non-negotiable. Fitness experts, who disagree about almost everything, are in agreement on this: *Without careful attention to diet, exercise is ineffective for fat loss.*

Read that again: **You absolutely, positively cannot lose appreciable amounts of fat without changing your diet.**

The standard argument for the final step in the fat-loss equation—exercise—is that it burns additional calories: It pads the "calories out" side of the standard "calories-in-calories-out" equation. Eat fewer calories while burning more calories and you're on

the road to a fitter you.

But some very striking 2016 research suggests that trying to burn a lot of additional calories to lose weight through exercise is... kind of futile.

The research, published in the *American Journal of Human Biology*, demonstrated convincingly that your body can only mobilize and burn so many calories per day. After you've burned through that allowance (running on the treadmill or lifting weights in the gym or planting geraniums in your garden), your body turns down your metabolic thermostat so that your net additional caloric burn is almost nil.

Long aerobic workouts can certainly have benefits. Within reason, your heart and lungs will thank you for extra time on the bike or on the road. But if your goal is burning extra fat, long workouts are impractical.

That's a hard one for most people to swallow, and the full picture is still taking shape. Most of us still think of food and exercise like matter and antimatter—one cancels the other out. But evolution has made the equation more complicated, capping the number of calories budgeted for exercise at just a few hundred per day. This is a concept called *adaptive thermogenesis*, and it may explain why your buddy who ran a marathon probably didn't lose much weight during training if he didn't also adjust his eating habits.

So the reason you exercise while trying to get leaner isn't to burn huge amounts of calories, but to send a simple message to your body: Keep the muscle and burn the fat. And you can send that message in way less time than it takes to burn 500 calories on a treadmill.

It takes about seven minutes.

Numerous studies have shown that if you diet without proper exercise, your body burns not just fat but a significant amount of muscle tissue as well. One study from 1999 compared two groups of adults following very low-calorie diets for 12 weeks, with one performing standard-issue cardio workouts, the other performing resistance-training workouts, like the ones in this book. Both groups lost weight—but the cardio group lost almost nine pounds of lean tissue in the process. The resistance trainers preserved all their muscle tissue.

A 2017 study found that older, obese adults who reduced their caloric intake but didn't exercise lost muscle tissue over a 10-week period. Those who followed the same diet, with additional protein and regular resistance training, however, preserved their muscle tissue over the same period.

So resistance training is vital. Without it, you're losing a ton of muscle tissue, which is a little like a CEO trying to cut costs by firing not just the slackers in the back room but her two most valuable workers as well.

Long-term, an exercise program built around solid workouts—like the ones in this book—fine-tunes your fat-burning metabolism. It grows muscle tissue and adds to the energy-producing mitochondria in those tissues. It improves your cardiovascular capacity, and it increases vascularization and circulation. It makes you more inclined to move throughout the rest of your day.

Forget the number of calories burned during your workout—these factors turn you into a better fat-burner, 24/7/365.

And that's your goal: not simply to burn calories but to re-jigger your entire metabolism so it's better at burning fat all the time. Cell by cell, workouts like the ones in this book turn you into a fat-burning beast, so that even if you fall off your diet—and life's too short not to do that from time to time—you won't balloon. The extra muscle you build gives you wiggle room so if you eat that chocolate cake at the wedding, or that bag of chips on the road trip, or that sundae on date night, your body can store that extra sugar in your newly built muscles as fuel for your next workout, rather than sock it away on your love handles to be burned off sometime in the late 2040s.

If you have a lot of weight to lose—say, 40 pounds or more—a seven-minute approach might work especially well. For one thing, if you're dieting intensely, you might simply not be up for long, involved workouts, especially if you have a stressful job, a family, a commute, and a pair of aging parents. Seven minutes might be just right to send that "burn fat, keep muscle" message without adding to the stress you're already shouldering.

And if you choose to do more than one seven-minute workout per day, as we recommend, you'll benefit by spiking your metabolism, sparking muscle growth, clearing blood sugar, and reducing stress many times a day—all of which contribute to further fat loss.

SEVEN-MINUTE WORKOUTS CAN HELP YOU MASTER CHALLENGING MOVEMENTS

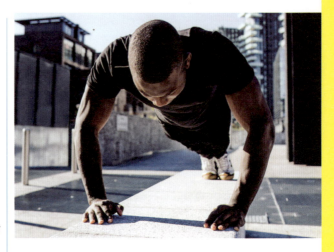

The toughest strength exercises—pushups, handstands, pullups, and other compound exercises— call on sometimes hundreds of joints and muscles with each rep. Such movements require not just muscle and strength but also skill: coordinated, balanced effort, distributed across your entire body. Elite powerlifters and strongmen— athletes who move more weight than anyone else on the planet—spend nearly as much time honing their technique in their various events as they do focusing on sheer strength and muscle.

Like riding a horse, playing the trumpet, or writing a legal brief, mastering challenging lifts takes repetition and practice. And much of that practice should be sub-maximal: well below a level of effort that seriously challenges your muscles. This is what Tsatsouline calls "greasing the groove," and it's undisputedly the best way to learn a new skill.

You've been "greasing the groove" yourself since you were an infant. Consider: When you learned to walk, you never worked to failure or felt the burn. You tried to walk for a few steps, toppled over, then repeated the process a few times. Then you got distracted, or sleepy, or hungry, and moved on to something else. When the mood struck you a few hours later, you tried again. And lo and behold, after a few weeks, you were walking like a champ: no tooth-gritting, no straining and cursing, no one yelling "It's all you!" in your dimpled face.

NFL quarterbacks work the same way. They don't practice Hail Marys until their throwing arms burn from the effort. They take breaks, tossing a few easy ones between big efforts, only throwing another long bomb when they're good and rested.

Lots of skill requires lots of rest.

If you're trying to master a tough bodyweight move, like an L-sit or the latest hand-stand challenge on TikTok, the best way to do it is to summon your inner child: Spread the effort out and avoid muscular failure like it's the coronavirus.

The seven-minute approach is the perfect approach for this type of low-stress, incremental movement toward mastery. Say, for example, you want to get better at pushups (and who doesn't?). The standard approach is to perform, say, three sets of about 12 reps. If you take each of those sets to failure, you'll likely be so sore you won't be able to think about doing pushups for two days or more. That's two days without practice—and two days when you're not getting better at pushups.

By performing shorter sets—well shy of failure—throughout your day, you avoid fatigue and breakdown, which allows you to get more meaningful practice reps in over time. So do six reps when you get up in the morning. Six more reps on your coffee break. Six more before lunch, six more after lunch, and so on. At the end of the day, you'll have accrued perhaps 50 reps—and you likely won't feel sore the next day.

Which means you can repeat the process and keep practicing.

When you push yourself to exhaustion, your technique suffers. Muscles don't

fire right. Balance and coordination head out the door. And at the end of your session, you're probably no closer to getting that full-range pullup or pushup than when you began.

In this book, you'll find skill-enhancing workouts that will help you conquer the toughest bodyweight moves. Trying to do the Superman pushup? The Quick-Interval Pushup Crusher, page 118, will get you there. Want high-skill moves for your upper and lower body? Take on High-Rep Muscle Mayhem, page 77, and Metabolic Interval Madness, page 79—but not on the same day.

Whatever fitness challenge you're trying to overcome, we've got you covered.

SEVEN-MINUTE WORKOUTS HELP YOU MOVE MORE

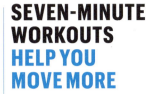

This one may sound insignificant: Isn't this a book about working out? Sweating, breathing heavy, building muscles? Stick with us: Moving around a little more may be the most crucial thing you can do for your health.

The benefits of walking, doing chores at home, and other forms of low-intensity movement have gotten a lot of play in the last few years—even to the point of becoming a national obsession with "getting your steps in."

Spoiler: There's nothing magical about that 10,000-step goal. That standard was dreamed up not by an exercise physiologist but by the makers of a Japanese pedometer in the 1960s. Still, those marketing geniuses got one thing right: There are serious health risks to sedentary living. Research has shown that the more time you spend sitting—working at a desk, commuting, and slouching over various screens—the higher your risk of health problems like heart disease, diabetes, and obesity.

So sitting around all day can lead to poor health—not terribly surprising.

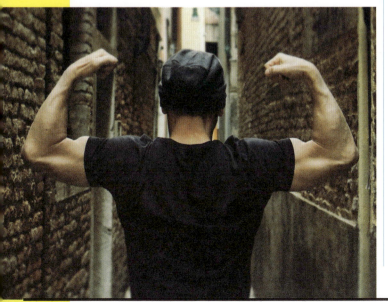

But here's the troubling kicker: The way we normally practice fitness—with an hour or so of intense, gym-based activity a few days a week—doesn't entirely mitigate the risks of an otherwise-sedentary life.

Let's take a hypothetical, 45-year-old gym-goer named Alonzo. Alonzo's a high-school math teacher, and he diligently hits the weights on Mondays, Wednesdays, and Fridays. Three other days a week, he does about an hour of cardio.

You'd think he'd have all his fitness boxes checked, right?

But then his doctor tells him his blood pressure is up, he's borderline diabetic, and he might have to start taking meds.

Bad luck? Awful genetics?

Hold on. Looking deeper at Alonzo's life, we see that he spends many hours a day reading, researching, and grading for his job. He commutes for another hour a day. And at night he sits on his couch, playing *Fortnite* and watching reruns of *Game of Thrones*, meditating on the many ways the final season could have been so much better.

Add it up, and Alonzo is parked in a chair 13 hours a day.

No matter how you slice it, that's a sedentary life. Even the most intense one-hour workout can't fully counterbalance the damage caused by 23 hours of virtual inactivity. Alonzo's workout sessions reduce his risk somewhat, but he'd likely be better off moving not only during his workouts, but more often throughout his day as well.

Researchers would say that Alonzo has plenty of EAT (exercise-activity thermogenesis, or energy burned during formal exercise) in his life, but very little NEAT (non-exercise activity thermogenesis— energy burned during other activities). And if you're trying to keep fat at bay, NEAT is an even bigger factor than formal exercise. Research suggests that NEAT is responsible for torching about 25 percent of the energy you burn in a day, as compared with exercise, which only burns about 5 to 10 percent of that energy. If you're looking to keep fat off and make your doctor happy, NEAT beats formal exercise every time.

Here's a few ways Alonzo might use seven-minute workouts to turn his troubling health indicators around. Instead of working out for an hour at a stretch, he might perform bite-sized workouts several times a day: once when he wakes up, once in the mid-morning, and so on. He's not adding any additional workout time to his life, but he's breaking up his sedentary time—which helps keep his blood pressure, and his blood sugar, down.

What if Alonzo loves his gym time? He craves the intensity and continuity of longer workouts. In that case, he might instead add a few workout snacks into his day on top of what he's already doing. Maybe he decides to focus on additional core or arm work, or up his mobility, or get better at pullups. With a few additional seven-minute sessions a week, Alonzo could make fast progress toward those fitness goals and drive his health risks way down.

Alternatively, Alonzo could combine the two approaches, performing a more standard 30-minute session in the morning and a few shorter workouts throughout the day.

And finally, Alonzo could do a mixture of all of the above, depending on what else he has going on that day.

Whichever approach he chooses, Alonzo is getting stronger, fitter, and healthier by including more movement throughout his day—a win not only for his physique but for his longevity and health as well.

FOUR COMMANDMENTS OF EATING FOR FAT LOSS

LIKE WE SAID BEFORE, you can't shed body fat without eating right. So to see results from the workouts you're about to do, you need to take your diet seriously. Consistency is king, and it's just as important to your nutrition as it is to your training. That doesn't mean you have to buy some elaborate meal plan subscription or eradicate all the joy from your dinner plate. In fact, the two key components of any successful diet (a caloric deficit and adequate protein consumption) are flexible enough that you shouldn't have to cut out entire foods from your life. Instead, all you need to do is focus on adding the right foods. When you fuel up strategically, you're less likely to

overdo it on snacks and sweets because you'll be full from all the good things you've already consumed. So what's your game plan? Let's break it down.

COMMANDMENT NO. 1
YOU NEED TO EAT MORE FOOD

If you have a Taco Bell Cheesy Gordita Crunch habit, the first step is easy: Limit your intake of anything with a name that includes the words "cheesy," "gordita," and/or "crunch."

But you still need to eat something, and whatever it is, it'll have calories you must account for. The accounting is

simple: There are two sides to the ledger. One side is your calorie intake, and the other is your metabolism—that is, the calories you burn—which works in four ways.

DIGEST. About 10 percent of your metabolism comes from how you process food. But you can do better if you eat more protein. That nutrient takes more energy to digest: 25 percent of protein calories are burned after you swallow them, compared with 2 to 3 percent of fat calories and 6 to 8 percent of calories from carbs.

MOVE. Everything from working out to walking to the mailbox burns more calories than not moving—and accounts for 20 to 30 percent of your metabolism. The more you move, the better, including those times when you...

HIT THE CAN. When you dial up a #1 or #2 (or sneak out a fart), energy leaves your body. Alas, you can't toot your way to single-digit body fat.

STAY ALIVE. The rest of the calories you eat go toward your body's other basic operating functions. (That's at least 60 percent of your metabolism.) By changing the "calories in" part of the formula, you also change the "calories out."

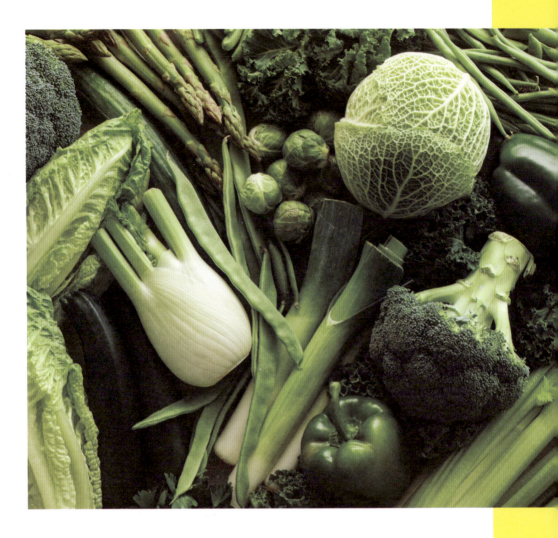

When you're putting less energy in the tank, you're likely to burn fewer calories during your workouts. That's the danger of cutting calories when you don't have a plan to maintain your new lower weight. Your metabolism slows, leaving you hungry and primed to regain the fat you lost, especially when hunger hits near a Taco Bell. The key is to reverse that process.

COMMANDMENT NO. 2
YOU NEED TO EAT BETTER FOOD

Pity the man forced to survive on gluten-free pizza and fat-free ice cream. Lucky for you, eating for fat loss requires you to eat real food. Here's the breakdown of your eating plan.

Eat 80 percent of your diet in whole and minimally processed foods that you like. "Whole" foods are ones that look like what they started out as: meat, fish, eggs, milk, nuts, seeds, fruits, vegetables, potatoes, and beans. One exception: protein powders. Sure, they're highly processed, but they're still a great way to consume the protein you need to make the plan work.

Eat 10 percent in whole and minimally processed foods that you don't necessarily like but don't hate (say, Swiss chard and lamb). This is intended to expand the range of nutrients you're eating. Maybe you'll even learn to like a new food, which means you're less likely to suffer from diet burnout.

Eat 10 percent in whatever the hell you want. Consider this your reward for faithfully embracing the two previous categories. Use this bonus however you'd like: Have a small indulgence every day, or save up for a bigger weekend junkfest. Even if it includes Cheesy Gordita Crunches.

Here's a shortcut: If the food doesn't have an ingredient list, it's a safe bet. Steak, apples, quinoa, eggplant, salmon—they're all single-ingredient foods. With packaged foods, each additional ingredient likely signals an extra step in processing, which may have stripped away some of the good stuff—including

tastiness. And often, to make up for lost flavor, food manufacturers pump processed foods with sugar and fat. These foods also tend to be higher in calories.

"Quality" also means taste. On this plan, you won't find any rules about foods you must eat. Nor will you find a list of foods you should never eat. Just about anything you already enjoy can fit into the plan, although perhaps not in the quantities you're used to eating.

COMMANDMENT NO. 3
MACRO-NUTRIENTS MATTER (ESPECIALLY PROTEIN)

Nutritionists refer to protein, carbs, and fat as "macros." Protein, of course, is the stuff of muscle growth, particularly branched-chain amino acids (BCAAs), including leucine. On our plan, you'll eat 1 gram of

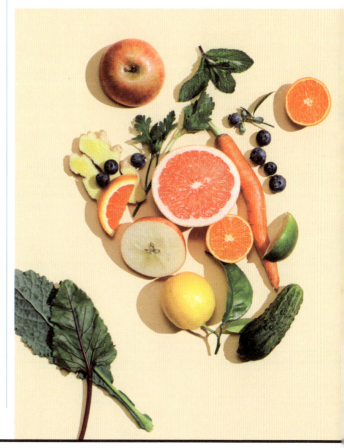

protein for every pound of your target body weight, or 25 percent to 35 percent of your daily diet.

But protein also increases satiation (feeling full at the end of a meal) and satiety (feeling less hungry between meals). So protein pulls triple duty: It speeds your metabolism, slows your appetite, and maintains muscle.

What about the other macros? For fat, you'll eat 0.4 to 0.7 gram of fat per pound of your target body weight per day. If you have a good chunk of body fat to lose, use the higher end of that scale, closer to 0.7. It's not that fat calories have any magical properties; a higher percentage of fat simply means fewer carbs. That tends to work better for heavier guys, who often are less sensitive to insulin, a hormone triggered by high-carbohydrate meals. Less sensitivity means more insulin; more insulin means your body will use less fat for energy. For everyone else, it's personal preference. For carbs, use any calories left over after you account for protein and fat. Who knew math could be so tasty?

COMMANDMENT NO. 4

MICRO-NUTRIENTS MATTER TOO

One risk of popular low-calorie diets: nutrient deficiency. That's because when you eat less food, it's harder to cover the basics. A multivitamin may help, but it probably won't contain enough immunity-fortifying magnesium or bone-building vitamin D. Research shows that eating a wide variety of foods provides the greatest benefit for overall health. To collect those key nutrients, dust off the old-fashioned idea of food groups.

Aim to include at least one food from each category every day, with some variety in fruits and vegetables, and you'll hit the full range of micronutrients you need to look good and feel great.

We know what you're thinking: What about my beer? Moderate drinking isn't likely to affect your weight in either direction as long as the calories from alcohol replace something else. If not, you'll probably gain fat. So swap out your carbs for alcohol. If you know you're going to have two beers out at the bar later, just eat 300 fewer carbohydrate calories (or 75 grams) that day.

So now that you understand the nutrition principles, it's time to learn how to use your seven-minute workouts to their fullest potential.

HERE'S YOUR MENU

- Meat and other protein-rich foods, including eggs and protein powder.

- Fat-rich foods, such as nuts and seeds, oil used for cooking or salad dressing, butter (and nut butters), olives, and avocados.

- Fibrous vegetables, including just about anything your mother said you had to eat if you wanted dessert.

- Starchy foods, such as grains (bread, cereal, pasta), legumes (beans and peas), and tubers (potatoes and other root vegetables).

- Milk and other dairy products, which includes all varieties of cheese, yogurt, and, yes, even chocolate milk.

- Fruits, fresh or dried. And no, Starbursts don't count.

HOW TO USE THIS BOOK

THERE ARE TWO major types of workouts in this book:

A **Total-Body Workout** covers all your major muscle groups in one session.

A **Muscle-Group Workout** focuses on a specific area in a single session.

There are also four **Recovery Workouts**, which we'll get into a little later.

There are about 625 muscles in your body, but to keep things simple, we're grouping all of the important ones into five major categories: your chest, back, legs, arms, and abs. Longtime fitness folks may complain that we're leaving some players out (hello, shoulders and glutes), but fear not: These workouts give all your skeletal muscles a thorough going-over.

At eight workouts per muscle group, this book features a total of 40 Muscle-Group Workouts—but just eight Total-Body Workouts. But

don't be fooled: Total-Body sessions and Muscle-Group sessions both play a vital role in your success.

THE CASE FOR TOTAL-BODY WORKOUTS

Total-Body Workouts are the ultimate in exercise efficiency. You fly through all your muscle groups lickety-split, then you're on with the rest of your day. The workouts are concentrated and fast, and, because you're placing a huge oxygen demand on many different muscles in sequence, you wind up getting a mini-cardio workout as well.

Total-Body Workouts closely resemble the kind of head-to-toe challenge that you get from playing sports—which is a big part of why we like them so much. It's great to look good, but it's even better if you also have the stamina and athleticism to use those muscles in the real world. Total-Body

Workouts teach you to do that.

And it's for all these reasons that, if you're pressed for time, Total-Body Workouts should form the backbone of your training schedule.

DOWNSIDE OF THE TOTAL-BODY APPROACH? The volume—that is, the total number of sets per muscle group—is fairly low. In seven minutes, you might perform just one or two sets for each major muscle group. That's good for basic strength and fitness, don't get us wrong, but it's on the low side if you're seeking more strength and muscle mass.

The solution is easy enough, though: Perform more than one session per workout day. That could be either more than one total-body scorcher, or a Total-Body Workout in conjunction with additional work for specific muscle groups—we'll show you how to do that below.

THE CASE FOR MUSCLE-GROUP WORKOUTS

Muscle-Group Workouts are focused and intense. Do them right, and after seven minutes, the working muscles will be completely torched. If you haven't experienced it before, you'll find there's something oddly satisfying about that feeling. You'll get a massive pump in your muscles, which feels cool and makes you look (temporarily) like you're visiting from the Marvel Universe. You also might feel a little sore for a day or two afterward—a strong indicator you've performed the exercises correctly and targeted the right muscle group. Score.

Volume—the raw number of hard sets you perform per muscle group—is definitely a factor in muscle growth, and Muscle-Group Workouts are a quick way to amp up those numbers fast. So if one of your priorities is building larger muscles, you should include at least some Muscle-Group Workouts in your workout week.

DOWNSIDE OF MUSCLE-GROUP WORKOUTS? They're inefficient. Building a full-body workout from Muscle-Group Workouts would take you 35 to 40 minutes (seven-minute workouts times five muscle groups plus a little time to catch your breath). Doable, but not ideal if speed and efficiency are of the essence.

For this reason, Muscle-Group Workouts aren't a good idea if you only have time for one workout a day. Do that, and you end up with a classic bro-split: chest on Monday, arms on Tuesday, back on Wednesday, and so on. It's your body, of course, but we don't much like

this approach: Even if you smoke your chest muscles with as many as three chest workouts on a Monday, you're not working them again for another week. That's like eating one huge meal once a week instead of three meals a day. You won't starve, but it's far from optimal.

This is why we recommend using Muscle-Group Workouts in conjunction with Total-Body Workouts for the best progress. The workouts are yours to mix and match, and are designed to stand on their own—but some ways of stacking them together work better than others.

Here are a few ideas on how to do that, based on your goals.

BEST FOR BEGINNERS

GOAL
Get in as much basic, balanced exercise as I can in as little time as possible.

SOLUTION
Do one Total-Body Workout a day, 3 to 7 times per week.

This is the simplest and most time-efficient approach, and it's great for beginners. Just grab a single Total-Body Workout and go for it. If you've never worked out before—or are coming off a layoff of six months or more—this method will give you some great gains: more strength, more muscle, more energy. If you choose this method, pick a different workout for each of the days you work out (so on Mondays you might do Total-Body Bodyweight Workout 1, on Wednesdays, Total-Body Weighted Workout 1, and Fridays, Total-Body Bodyweight Workout 2, then repeat the sequence the following week). You'll hit all your muscles each

time you work out, so nothing gets lost in the shuffle. If you happen to miss a workout now and again, no big deal: You'll make up for it on your next workout day.

Just starting out? You might want to work up to the seven-day version over a few weeks. Conventional wisdom holds that you shouldn't work out two days in a row—but if you're doing different workouts, and therefore different exercises—each day you work out, you should be fine.

Here's a sample of how you might put your workout week together:

MONDAY	TUESDAY	WEDNESDAY	THURSDAY	FRIDAY	SATURDAY	SUNDAY
Total-Body Workout	Rest	Total-Body Workout	Rest	Total-Body Workout	Rest	Rest

THE MINIMALIST TWO-A-DAY APPROACH

GOAL
Get my exercise in, and add some additional muscle in the process.

SOLUTION
Do a Total-Body Workout in the morning and a Muscle-Group Workout in the evening, 3 to 7 times per week.

For people with a little more time who want an additional challenge, this is a great option: Power through one seven-minute session before work, then another one later in the day.

One way to approach this system is to stick with full-body sessions in the morning, then do a Muscle-Group Workout in the afternoon or evening: a back workout, a leg workout, or any other area you think needs additional attention.

Below is one way of scheduling your workout week with these parameters:

	MONDAY	TUESDAY	WEDNESDAY	THURSDAY	FRIDAY	SATURDAY	SUNDAY
AM	Total-Body Workout	Rest	Total-Body Workout	Rest	Total-Body Workout	Rest	Rest
PM	Legs Workout	Chest Workout	Abs Workout	Back Workout	Arms Workout	Rest	Rest

Note: In this schedule, you're working your whole body three times a week in the mornings, and performing individual Muscle-Group Workouts five times a week.

THE ULTIMATE FAT-LOSS STRATEGY

GOAL
Lose maximum amount of fat.

SOLUTION
Perform Total-Body Workout "snacks" frequently throughout your day; on alternate days, perform Muscle-Group Workouts. The first day you do this, do a leg workout and a chest workout. The second day, do a leg workout and a back workout.

When the goal is losing as much fat as you can, you want to work as much muscle mass per workout as possible. Since 60 percent of your muscle mass is in your legs, that's where your efforts will focus: waist down.

Don't worry, though: Your arms, torso, and core will still get plenty of work so as you burn the fat off, you'll have something to show underneath.

A sample week might look like this:

	MONDAY	TUESDAY	WEDNESDAY	THURSDAY	FRIDAY	SATURDAY	SUNDAY
AM	Total-Body Workout	Legs Workout	Total-Body Workout	Legs Workout	Total-Body Workout	Rest	Rest
MID	Total-Body Workout	Rest	Abs Workout	Rest	Total-Body Workout	Rest	Rest
PM	Total-Body Workout	Chest Workout, Abs Workout	Total-Body Workout	Back Workout, Arms Workout	Total-Body Workout	Rest	Rest

THE MUSCLE-BUILDING PLAN

GOAL
Build maximum muscle and strength.

SOLUTION
Perform Upper Body and Lower Body Workouts on alternate days

To stimulate growth, you want to work each muscle as hard as possible—which means workouts that focus on individual muscle groups. This is as close as we think you should get to the bro-split: dividing the body into two major areas and blasting them on alternate days.

There are a lot of ways to organize this, but we like a "four-days-on, one-day-off" rotation, where you have two different workout days—call them A and B—which you perform alternately. In all but your Arms and Abs workouts,

you have the choice to perform one, two, or three workouts. You can stick with the same circuit on each round or mix it up as you wish.

WORKOUT DAY A:
Chest Workout (1–3/day);
Back Workout (1–3/day)

WORKOUT DAY B:
Legs Workout (1–3/day);
Arms Workout, Abs Workout

Every two rotations, you take a rest day. So if you're starting your workouts on a Monday, your first two weeks would look like this:

	MONDAY	TUESDAY	WEDNESDAY	THURSDAY	FRIDAY	SATURDAY	SUNDAY
WK 1	Workout A	Workout B	Workout A	Workout B	Rest	Workout A	Workout B
WK 2	Workout A	Workout B	Rest	Workout A	Workout B	Workout A	Workout B

Note: Since you've just completed four days of workouts, you'd begin the following Monday with a well-earned rest day. Note that the workouts don't correspond to the days of the week in this schedule: Depending on where you are in the schedule, any day could wind up an A day, a B day, or a rest day. Miss a day? Just pick up the rotation where you left off.

This approach gives your muscles plenty of stimulation—and stress. So don't take it on unless you have time and energy to recover from it. Feel free to divide your workouts into morning and evening sessions here as well— i.e., on an A day, you could work your chest in the morning and your back in the evening.

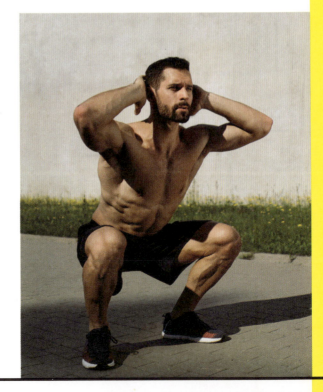

THE CONSTANT SHAKE-UP STRATEGY

GOAL
Stay fit and don't get bored.

SOLUTION
Three total-body workouts per week—plus anything that strikes your fancy (within limits).

Like to shake things up? Not big on structure? We get it: Not everyone lives and dies by their pullup numbers, and many people feel their days are scheduled and structured enough as it is. If you just bought this book to make things easy and fun, that's cool too.

In that case, we still recommend at least three Total-Body Workouts per week on nonconsecutive days: You'll hit every muscle, get a little cardio work in, and stave off chronic disease. There's eight Total-Body Workouts in the book: Feel free to mix 'em up.

But that's only 21 minutes of your life. Any other time the mood grabs you, go crazy. Open to a random page and go for it. Or work through the book sequentially.

The one caveat: Don't perform a Muscle-Group Workout for the same area two days in a row. Those workouts require about 48 hours of rest before you repeat them. So you don't want to do, say, a Total-Body Workout on Monday morning and a chest workout Monday evening—wait until at least Wednesday before doing another chest workout.

	MONDAY	TUESDAY	WEDNESDAY	THURSDAY	FRIDAY	SATURDAY	SUNDAY
AM	Rest	Legs Workout	Total-Body Workout	Rest	Rest	Rest	Rest
PM	Arms Workout	Rest	Rest	Back Workout, Arms Workout	Rest	Total-Body Workout	Rest

HOW TO USE THE RECOVERY WORKOUTS

As noted, this book also includes four Recovery Workouts. We admit that sounds a little contradictory: How can you recover doing more of the very thing that made you sore in the first place?

Stick with us: Recovery Workouts consist mostly of easy stretches and light, circulation-boosting movement. When you're sore, stiff, and tired, there's no better solution than this type of movement to ease the pain and help you rejuvenate. You'll increase circulation to those stiff and tired areas, pushing oxygenated blood into them and driving CO_2 out. You'll activate the muscles that stabilize your joints and keep your spine safe. And you'll restore range of motion in areas where the surrounding muscles are tight and sore.

You can do Recovery Workouts any time. When you wake up, midday, before you go to bed. Do them while you're watching TV, or waiting in line at the grocery store. If you're particularly sore or tired, sub a Recovery Workout in for a regular workout.

Once you see how good you feel doing Recovery Workouts—and how much they help your performance in your regular workouts—you won't want to stop.

WHEN TO CHANGE THINGS UP

So you've got some marching orders: a rough idea of where to start and how to structure your workout week.

Should you just do that forever?

No. Even the absolute best workout program, performed with spot-on form and perfect recovery, only works for eight weeks, at the outside. And the more experienced you are, the sooner a workout program becomes ineffective. We've all known folks who do the same workout schedule for years. They don't lose much ground, but they don't get much fitter, and they're not very engaged or inspired, either.

The flip side, however, is the program-hopper who changes their workout program every week: one week it's Pilates, the next it's powerlifting, the next thing you know they've signed up for a triathlon.

There's value in both consistency and experimentation, but for optimal progress you need a balance of both.

So we suggest changing things up about every month or so.

With 52 workouts to work with, you can easily sub out one Arms Workout or Recovery Workout or Total-Body Workout for another

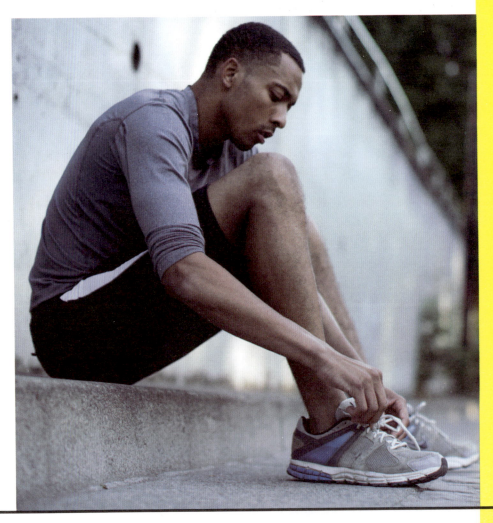

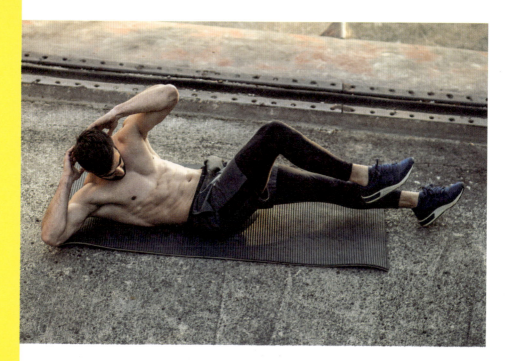

one from the same category—and that means you can stick with a workout program with the same basic structure, while still including plenty of variation.

Or you can take a more radical approach and change the entire structure of your program, based either on a new set of priorities, the recommendations above, or your own curiosity.

WEIGHTS OR NO WEIGHTS?

Trainers love to argue about the best exercises, the best equipment, the best workouts.

Among their favorite points of contention: What's better—workouts with or without weights?

In truth, the question itself is flawed: A weight is a tool. Ask a carpenter whether a saw or a hammer is better, and you'd be met with a quizzical look: Both are essential for carpentry. Which one you use depends on the context.

So we like both strategies: Bodyweight moves are the ultimate in convenience and accessibility, while dumbbells offer greater variety and ease of scalability. Both types of movements give you something a little different, and variety is something your muscles and nervous system really, really like. So don't choose between them: Get

some adjustable weights (ideally going up to at least 25 pounds to start), and use them in conjunction with bodyweight exercises when you're home. On the road? No need to skimp on your workouts: You've got a whole sea of bodyweight moves, and workouts, to choose from.

On the subject of weight: choosing the amount of resistance to use on any given exercise is half-science, half-art.

Ideally you want a weight that allows you to perform the number of reps assigned in the workout—but just barely. So if a workout says to perform three sets of 15 reps on a given exercise, you want all three sets to be tough, and on that final set, you should be in serious doubt as to whether you can complete all 15 reps at all. If you do, increase the resistance on that exercise next time you perform that workout.

Working to failure—that is, momentary exhaustion of the working muscle group—is a much-debated topic. Current research suggests that it's not necessary for muscles to grow, and that you can do just as well stopping each set a rep or two shy of failure.

Generally speaking, that's good advice. But if you never hit the wall on an exercise—never reach the point where you can't go on, even with a supreme effort—you'll never really know how strong you are. Even longtime fitness vets surprise themselves when they work to 100 percent failure: they often find they had five, seven, or even 10 reps in the tank when they thought they were stopping one or two reps from failure.

Our advice: work hard on all your sets, reaching failure—or close to it—on your last set of most exercises.

FINAL NOTE: WORK HARD (BUT DON'T DO ANYTHING THAT HURTS)

We've heard many a smart coach say *a training program is only as good as the effort you put into it.* If you work hard at it, a poorly designed program will get much better results than a brilliantly designed one that you half-ass your way through.

This book contains 52 workouts created by experts that absolutely will deliver results—if you do them properly and work hard.

None of them will do you much good if you don't push yourself a little: Work till your muscles burn, get a little sore the next day, emit the occasional grunt. Workout vets learn to expect and even, perversely, enjoy that sensation, knowing that they're getting stronger and spurring new growth. Asked how many situps he did, Muhammad Ali once quipped, "I don't start counting till it hurts." Like any gym vet, The Greatest knew that it's those at-your-edge reps that count.

There's a flip side of that argument, however: Pain for pain's sake is never the goal. Way too often, we see folks at the gym take foolish risks using weights they can't control, compromising their form, and risking serious injury. You probably have, too. They've taken the "push yourself" advice much too far.

The people who make the best progress—and we really, really want you to become one of them—are sticklers for form. Every rep looks like something you'd see in a textbook. Their backs are straight, their hips and shoulders are aligned. They're feeling their way through every rep of every set, making sure that their mechanics are perfect and the right muscles are doing the brunt of the work. Their workouts are focused, precise, and effective—but the second they feel something "off"—the burning in their muscles wanders into their joints, their back, neck, or some other vulnerable area—they terminate the set immediately.

Learning to work out with that kind of precision takes time, no less than becoming a great golfer or writer or piano player—or doing much of anything worthwhile. Everyone who contributed to this book is a lifer, and all of us strive daily to dial in our exercise form ever more precisely. Some days we hit it, and we feel great. Other days we might push too hard—or not hard enough. But we regroup, rest, recharge, and get after it the next day, determined to do more with better form.

We hope you'll join us on this quest. It's a worthy one.

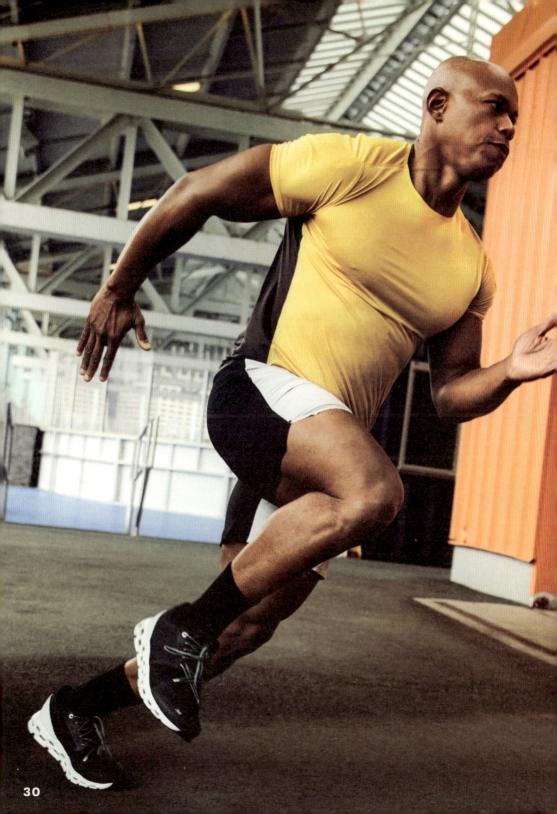

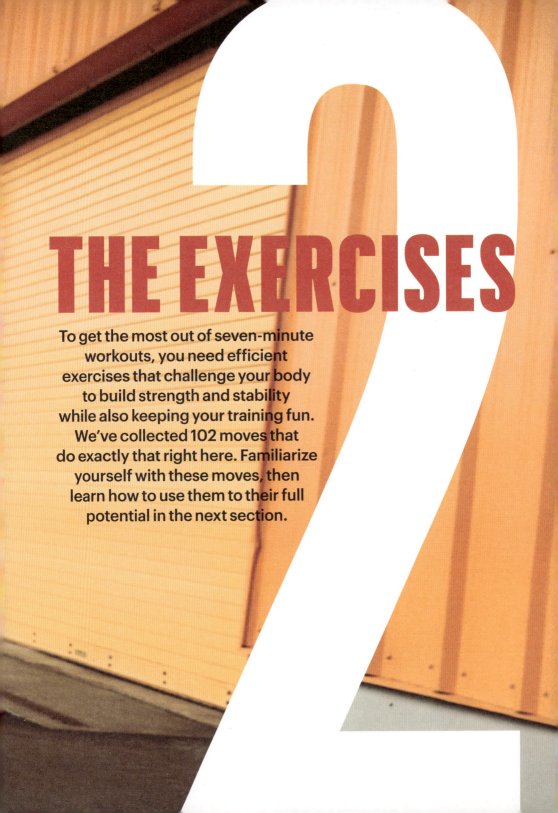

THE EXERCISES

To get the most out of seven-minute workouts, you need efficient exercises that challenge your body to build strength and stability while also keeping your training fun. We've collected 102 moves that do exactly that right here. Familiarize yourself with these moves, then learn how to use them to their full potential in the next section.

2

BODYWEIGHT – ABS

BEAR CRAWL

▶ Get on all fours, hands under shoulders and knees under hips. Lift your knees off the floor so only your hands and toes are touching the floor. Moving your opposite hands and feet together (left hand and right foot, right hand and left foot), crawl forward. Continue for the prescribed amount of time.

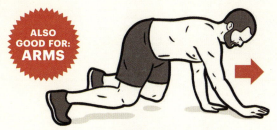

ALSO GOOD FOR: **ARMS**

BEAR REVERSE CRAWL

▶ Position yourself on the floor on your hands and knees. Hands should be directly below your shoulders and knees should be directly below your hips, feet flexed.

▶ Dig your toes into the floor, press your hands into the floor, and lift your knees 1 inch off the floor. Lift your right arm and left leg, move both limbs 3 inches backward, and return them to the floor. Repeat with your left arm and right leg to continue to crawl in reverse. Continue for the prescribed amount of time.

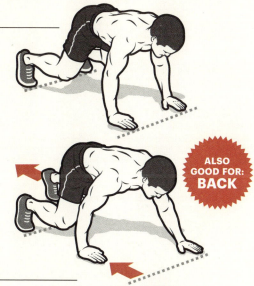

ALSO GOOD FOR: **BACK**

BEAST TAP

▶ Position yourself on the floor on your hands and knees, hands directly below your shoulders and knees directly below your hips, feet flexed.

▶ Dig your toes into the floor, press your hands into the floor, and lift your knees 1 inch. Contract your abs and lift one hand off the floor, then tap the opposite shoulder while maintaining a strong spinal position. Return your hand to the floor and repeat on the opposite side. That's 1 rep. Perform the specified number of reps.

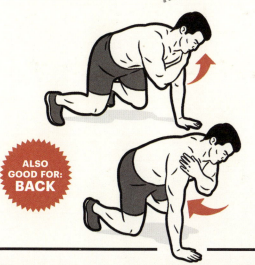

ALSO GOOD FOR: **BACK**

BEAST BOX DRILL

▶ Position yourself on the floor on your hands and knees. Your hands should be directly below your shoulders and your knees should be directly below your hips, feet flexed.

▶ Dig your toes into the floor, press your hands into the floor, and lift your knees 1 inch off the floor. Lift your right arm and left leg, move both limbs 3 inches forward, then put them back on the floor. Then take 2 steps to the left, 2 backward, and 2 to the right, creating a box. Make sure to work both clockwise and counter-clockwise. Continue for the prescribed amount of time.

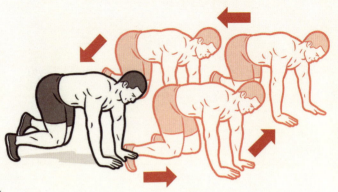

BICYCLE CRUNCH

▶ Lying on your back, hands behind your head and elbows out, raise your legs and move them as if cycling. Lift your head and shoulders off the floor as you bicycle, then lower them. Continue for the prescribed amount of time.

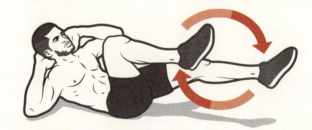

BODYWEIGHT WIPER

▶ Lie on your back with your legs extended straight up and perpendicular to the floor. Lower your legs to the floor, keeping them straight. Reverse the move to return to the starting position. Repeat on the opposite side. Continue alternating back and forth for the prescribed time.

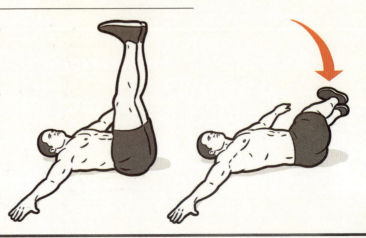

BODYWEIGHT – ABS

CRAB GRAB

▶ Assume a crab-walk position with your heels beneath your knees and your palms beneath your shoulders. Lift your hips, raise your right hand and left leg over your torso, and try to grab your toes. Return to the starting position. Repeat with your left hand and right leg. That's 1 rep.

ALSO GOOD FOR: BACK

DEADBUG

▶ Lie on your back on the floor. Contract your abs and drive your lower back into the floor to create a strong lower back position. The goal is to eliminate any space between your back and the floor. Not even a pencil should fit between. Raise your legs so your hips and knees are bent at 90-degree angles, and extend your arms overhead, perpendicular to the floor.

▶ Focus on holding this position, and extend one leg and the opposite arm. Extend only as far as you can without losing that back-to-the-floor position. Use your abs and hips to maintain the lower back position. If you begin arching your back, you may be overextending your shoulders. Keep fighting to keep your lower back grounded; it's OK if your arm stays above the floor. After you've moved all four limbs, that's 1 rep.

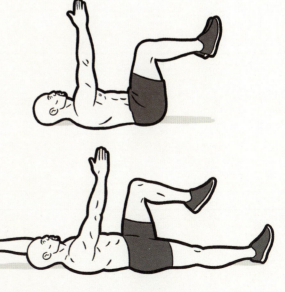

HOLLOW BODY CRUNCH ROCK

▶ Lie flat on your back with your legs stretched out and arms extended directly overhead. Lift your legs 6 inches off the floor then lift your upper body so your shoulder blades are no longer in contact with the floor.

▶ Engage your core by bending your knees and elbows and pulling them in to meet above your waistline. Rock here for 3 seconds. From this contracted position, slowly extend your limbs out to return to the starting position. That's 1 rep. Continue for the prescribed number of reps.

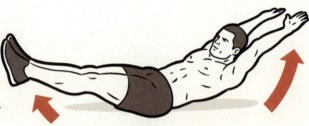

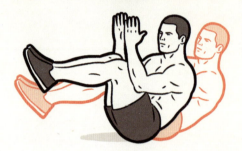

HOLLOW HOLD

▶ Lie on your back, arms and legs tucked. Tighten your abs, pressing your lower back into the floor. Then extend your legs as far as you can while continuing to press your lower back into the ground. Extend your arms as far overhead as you can. Hold for the prescribed amount of time.

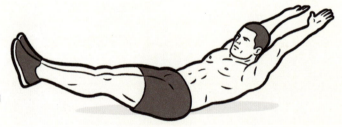

VARIATION
WEIGHTED HOLLOW HOLD

▶ Perform Hollow Hold as described above, but hold a dumbbell in each hand.

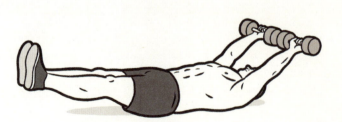

BODYWEIGHT – ABS

LYING DUMBBELL LEG LIFT

▶ Lie on your back, holding a light dumbbell between your feet.

▶ Extend your arms overhead to form a Y, or keep them by your sides. Squeeze your abs, pull your ribs in tight, and press your lower back close to the floor. Maintain this tension throughout the movement.

▶ Keeping your legs as straight as possible, raise them until they are just short of 90 degrees to the floor. Hold for a moment, then lower legs until your feet are about 3 inches above the floor. That's 1 rep.

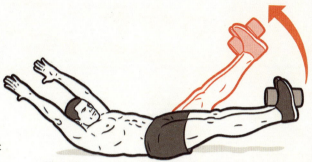

PLANK

▶ Get into a pushup position with your hands slightly wider than your shoulders. Engage your abs and glutes to create a straight line from your shoulders to your ankles. Hold for the prescribed amount of time.

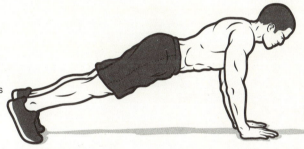

PLANK JACK

▶ Get into a pushup position, then bend your elbows to lower your forearms until they're resting on the floor. Your elbows should be in line with your shoulders, and your body should form a straight line, head to feet. Jump your feet out to each side as if you were doing a jumping jack, landing on the balls of your feet. Jump your feet back in. That's 1 rep. Repeat for prescribed amount of time.

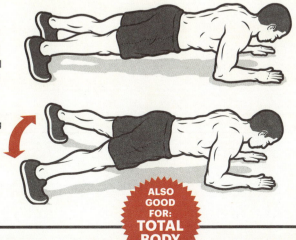

ALSO GOOD FOR: **TOTAL BODY**

PLANK WITH KNEE TO ELBOW

▶ Start in a high-plank position—a.k.a. the pushup position. Lift your right foot off the floor and draw your knee up to your right elbow, keeping your body straight from shoulders to ankles. Pause for a moment, then return to the start. Repeat on the left side. Continue for the prescribed amount of time.

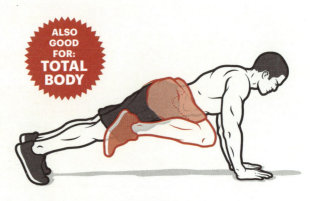

ALSO GOOD FOR: **TOTAL BODY**

PLANK WITH LEG LIFT

▶ Assume a pushup position but with your weight on your forearms instead of your hands. Brace your abs, clench your glutes, and keep your body straight from head to heels.

▶ Now raise your right leg and hold that position for 1 second. Lower your right leg and raise your left leg. That's 1 rep. Continue alternating back and forth for the prescribed time or reps.

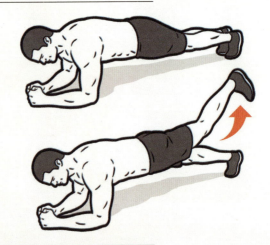

REVERSE CRUNCH

▶ Lie faceup on the floor with your arms by your sides, palms facing down. Bend your hips and knees 90 degrees.

▶ Raise your hips off the floor and crunch them inward toward your chest. Pause, then slowly lower your legs until your heels nearly touch the floor. That's 1 rep.

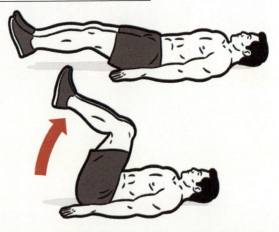

BODYWEIGHT – ABS

SHOULDER TAP

▶ Start in a pushup or high plank position with your shoulders directly above your hands. Your feet should be approximately shoulder-width apart. Squeeze your glutes and your abs as tight as possible to create total-body tension.

▶ From this firm position, bring your right hand up and tap your left shoulder, then return it to its original position. Next, bring your left hand up and tap your right shoulder, then place it back in its original position. That's 1 rep.

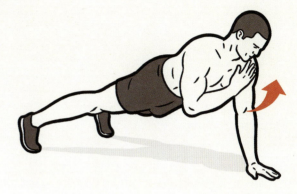

SIDE PLANK

▶ Lie on your right side, legs straight. Squeeze your abs and prop yourself up on your right forearm, creating a straight line from shoulders to feet. Hold for the prescribed amount of time.

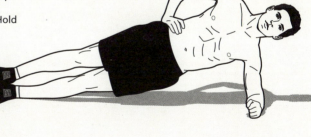

SIDE PLANK OVER AND BACK

▶ Lie on your side with your elbow planted on the floor directly below your shoulder. Scissor your feet, with the top foot forward and the bottom foot behind.

▶ Engage your abs and glutes to maintain a stable line from shoulders to hips to feet, and lift your front leg off the floor. Then swing it back and tap your foot behind your bottom leg. Slowly return the front foot back to the starting position. That's 1 rep. Continue for the prescribed number of reps.

SIDE PLANK WITH TOP ARM REACH

▶ Assume a side plank position on your right side: feet stacked, right hand and forearm on the floor, and your body straight from your head to your heels. Extend your left arm directly upward, fingers spread wide, palm facing forward. This is your starting position.

▶ Maintaining the plank position, reach your left hand down and underneath your torso as far as you can.

▶ Reverse the move and return to the starting position. That's 1 rep.

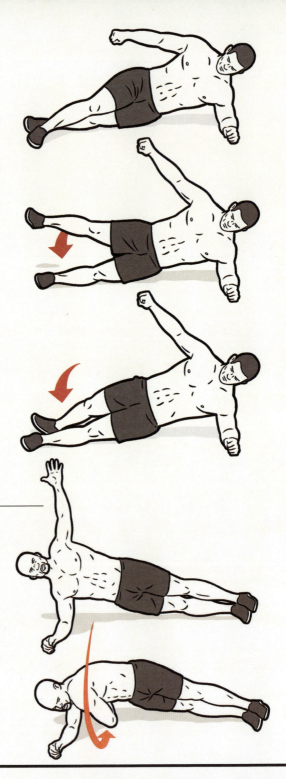

BODYWEIGHT – ABS

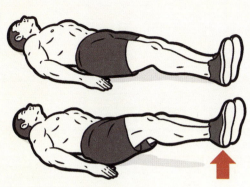

SUPINE LEG LIFT

▶ Lie on your back on the floor with your legs extended and arms at your sides.

▶ Lift your legs 6 inches off the floor while maintaining tension in your core and legs. Hold for a moment, then release. That's 1 rep.

V-UP

▶ Lie on your back with your legs straight and together and your arms extended past your head and in line with your body.

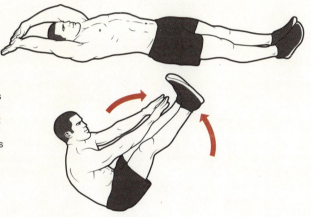

▶ In one movement, simultaneously lift your upper body and your legs as if you're trying to touch your fingers to your toes; you'll be balanced on your sit bones. Keep your legs straight and your head in line with your torso. Your body should form a V. Lower arms and legs back to starting position. That's 1 rep. You can also perform V-Ups with dumbbells, holding light weights in each hand.

3-POINT BEAST

▶ Position yourself on the floor on your hands and knees. Your hands should be directly below your shoulders, your knees should be directly below your hips, and your feet should be flexed.

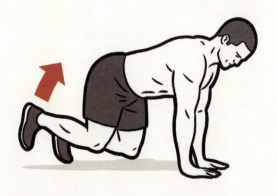

▶ Dig your toes into the floor, press your hands into the floor, and elevate your knees 1 inch. Then lift one of your limbs 1 or 2 inches off the floor, hold it for a second, then return it to the floor. Try to maintain your stability, and continue until you've lifted each limb 1 time. That's 1 rep. Repeat for the prescribed number of reps.

BODYWEIGHT – **ARMS**

CLOSE-GRIP PUSHUP

▶ Assume a pushup position, but keep your hands directly under your elbows. Keeping your elbows as close to your torso as possible and your core tight, lower your chest to the floor; push back up. Repeat for the prescribed amount of time.

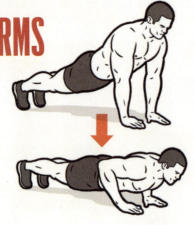

CLOSE-GRIP T-STOP PUSHUP

▶ Get into the pushup position, hands on the floor slightly narrower than shoulder-width.

▶ Keeping your body straight and your elbows close to your sides, lower your chest all the way to the floor. Release your grip and extend your arms directly outward, palms down.

▶ Return your hands to the pushup position. Keeping your body straight, push yourself back up to the starting position. That's 1 rep. Repeat as prescribed in the workout.

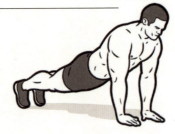

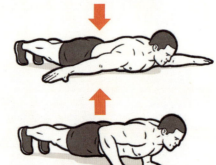

HANDS-ELEVATED CLOSE-GRIP PUSHUP

▶ Perform a close-grip pushup as described above but with your hands on a bench or other other elevated surface (a coffee table or kitchen counter will do). Do a pushup, bringing your chest to touch the bench at the bottom of each rep. One pushup is 1 rep.

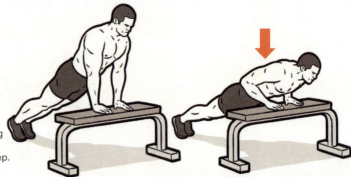

BODYWEIGHT – **ARMS**

ISO TRICEPS SQUEEZE

▶ Stand upright, arms at your sides.

▶ Make fists with your hands and extend your arms down and back as hard as you can, squeezing the backs of your upper arms as hard as possible. Hold until time is up.

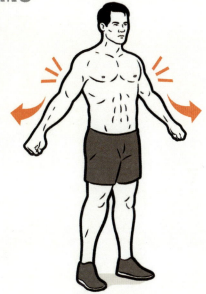

FRENCH PRESS PUSHUP

▶ Get into a pushup position, hands shoulder-width apart and under your shoulders. Walk your hands about 6 inches forward. Your arms will be angled from the floor to your torso.

▶ Keeping your body straight and your forearms parallel, slowly lower your elbows until they are 1 to 3 inches from the floor. Don't let your elbows flare out.

▶ Quickly reverse the move and return to the starting position. That's 1 rep.

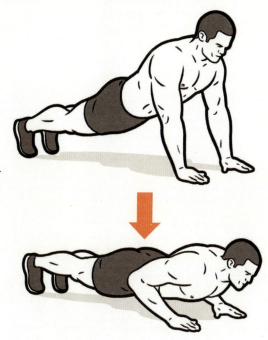

BODYWEIGHT – **BACK**

BENT-OVER W

▶ Start bent at the hips, arms hanging. Lift your arms to your sides, elbows bent, forearms angled up 45 degrees to form a W; then lower them. That's 1 rep. Repeat for the prescribed number of reps.

BENT-OVER T

▶ Start bent at the hips, arms hanging. Raise your arms straight out to your sides to form a T; then lower them. That's 1 rep. Repeat for the prescribed number of reps.

BENT-OVER Y

▶ Stand straight, then bend at the hips and push your butt back until your torso is at a 30-degree angle with the floor. Let your arms hang. Now raise your arms overhead to form a Y; then lower them. That's 1 rep. Repeat for the prescribed number of reps.

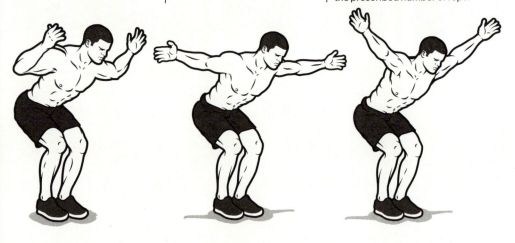

RAG DOLL

▶ Stand upright with knees slightly bent. Hinge forward at the hips, letting your head and arms hang from your waist, grasping each elbow with the opposite hand. Hold for the prescribed amount of time.

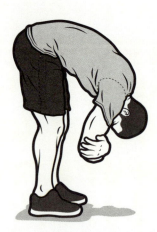

BODYWEIGHT – BACK

REVERSE T-RAISE

▶ Lie facedown with your arms extended straight out from your shoulders so your body forms a T. Make a fist, thumbs pointing upward and palms forward; your pinky fingers will be contacting the floor.

▶ Raise your arms directly upward, squeezing your shoulder blades together and contracting the backs of your shoulders (deltoids).

▶ Hold for one count, then slowly return to the starting position. That's 1 rep.

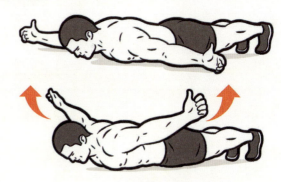

SCAPULAR RETRACTION

▶ Extend your arms at shoulder height and place your hands slightly wider than shoulder-width apart on a wall. Keeping your elbows as straight as you can, squeeze your shoulder blades together to move your torso closer to the wall. Hold for the prescribed amount of time. Release to starting position.

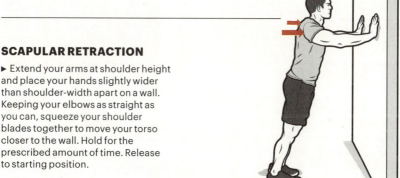

SUPERMAN

▶ Lie on your belly with your legs and arms fully extended, like Superman in flight. Your palms and the tops of your feet should be flat on the floor.

▶ Engage your glutes and back extensors to lift your legs and upper body (shoulders and pecs) off the floor. Hold for 3 seconds, then gently lower back to the floor. That's 1 rep.

VARIATION
SUPERMAN WITH WEIGHTS

▶ Perform Superman as described above, but hold a light dumbbell in each hand.

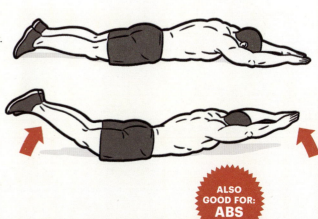

ALSO GOOD FOR: ABS

BODYWEIGHT – CHEST

DEADSTOP PUSHUP

▶ Assume a pushup position with your feet together, your body straight, and your hands below but slightly wider than your shoulders. Lower your body all the way to the floor. Lift your hands, pause, and then place them back on the floor and push up explosively.

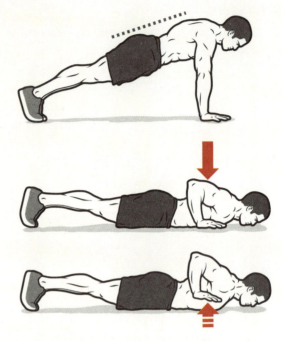

HANDS-ELEVATED PUSHUP

▶ Put your hands slightly wider than shoulder-width apart on a bench or other other elevated surface (a coffee table or kitchen counter will do). Do a pushup, bringing your chest to touch the bench at the bottom of each rep. One pushup is 1 rep.

BODYWEIGHT – CHEST

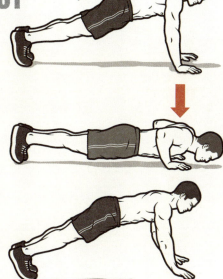

PLYO PUSHUP

▶ Assume a pushup position with your feet together, arms straight, and hands slightly wider than your shoulders. Lower your body to the floor, and then push up with enough force for your hands to leave the floor. Land and repeat for the prescribed amount of time.

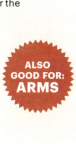

ALSO GOOD FOR: **ARMS**

PUSHUP

▶ Start in the plank position, core tight and glutes squeezed, hands directly below your shoulders. Bend at the elbows and shoulders, lowering your torso until your chest is an inch from the floor. Pause, then push back up. That's 1 rep. Repeat for prescribed number of reps.

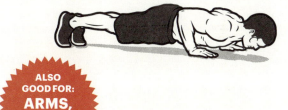

ALSO GOOD FOR: **ARMS, TOTAL BODY**

T-STOP PUSHUP

▶ Start in a plank position, arms extended. Do a pushup, then lower yourself completely to the floor. Throw your hands out to your sides. Return hands to starting position and push up. That's 1 rep. Perform for the prescribed amount of time.

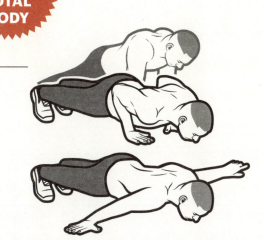

BODYWEIGHT – LEGS

180-DEGREE JUMP

▶ Start in an athletic stance, then drop your weight slightly and swing your arms behind you. Quickly reverse the movement, swinging your arms overhead and jumping as high as you can, simultaneously spinning your body clockwise 180 degrees.

▶ Land softly and repeat, this time spinning the opposite direction. That's 1 rep.

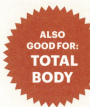

ALSO GOOD FOR:
TOTAL BODY

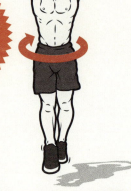

ALTERNATING LUNGE

▶ Stand tall, arms at your sides, core engaged. Step your right leg forward into a lunge, lowering your left knee to the floor. Return to starting position. Repeat on the left side and continue for the prescribed amount of time.

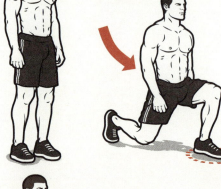

BODYWEIGHT SQUAT

▶ Stand as tall as you can, feet shoulder-width apart, and hold your arms straight out in front of your chest. Push your hips back and lower your body until your thighs are at least parallel to the floor. Drive back up to the starting position. Repeat as quickly as you can for the prescribed amount of time.

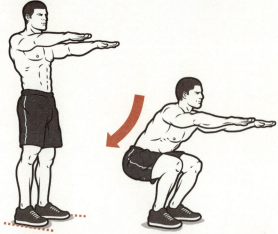

BODYWEIGHT – LEGS

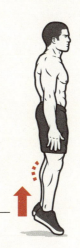

CALF RAISE

▶ Stand in a relaxed position and rise up high on your toes, going as high as you can; you'll feel a contraction in your calf muscles. Hold for 2 seconds, then lower. That's 1 rep.

HIP HINGE

▶ Stand tall, arms at your sides. Putting your weight in your heels, push your butt back; you might feel the muscles and tendons around your hamstrings and glutes activate and stretch. For more activation, push your butt further out. If your toes come up, that's fine. Hold for the prescribed amount of time.

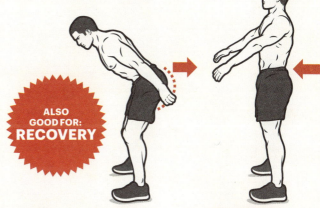

ALSO GOOD FOR: RECOVERY

INCHWORM TO RUNNER'S STRETCH

▶ Bend at the waist and touch the floor, then walk your hands out until you're in a pushup position. Step your right foot forward, outside your right hand. Lift your right hand and reach up, arm straight. Return to the pushup position and reverse the move back to standing. Repeat on the left side. That's 1 rep.

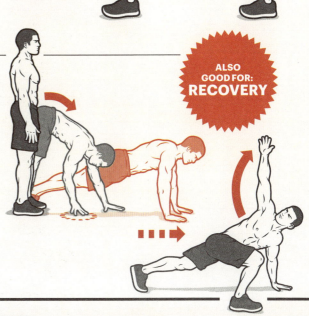

ALSO GOOD FOR: RECOVERY

JUMP SQUAT

▶ Stand up straight, then lower your torso until your thighs are parallel to the floor. Then jump as high as you can. After you land, immediately launch your next jump. Repeat for prescribed number of reps or amount of time.

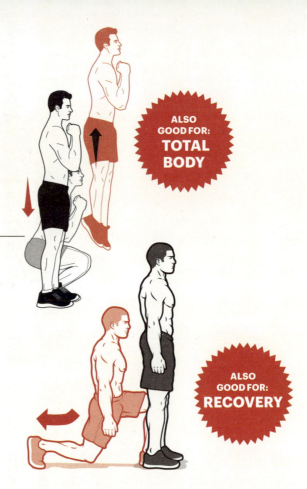

ALSO GOOD FOR: TOTAL BODY

REVERSE LUNGE

▶ Stand tall, arms at your sides, core engaged. Step your right leg back into a reverse lunge, lowering your knee to the floor. Step back far enough that you feel a stretch in your right hip. Return to starting position. That's 1 rep.

VARIATION
ALTERNATING REVERSE LUNGE

▶ Perform reverse lunge as described but alternate legs. One lunge on each leg equals 1 rep.

ALSO GOOD FOR: RECOVERY

SHIN BOX TO TALL KNEELING

▶ Sit on your butt on the floor with your knees in front of you, bent at 90 degrees. Keep your heels on the floor and raise your toes.

▶ Maintain an upright position and shift both legs to the left until the outside of your left knee and inside of your right knee are on the floor. Extend your hips up, shifting your body into a tall, upright position—use your arms for balance and keep your core tight. Hold this position for 2 seconds. Slowly descend back to the floor and repeat in the opposite direction. After you've shifted to both sides, you've done 1 rep. Repeat for prescribed number of reps.

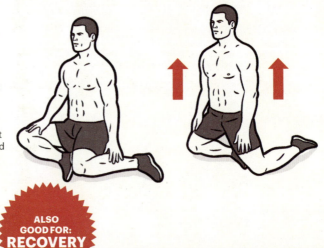

ALSO GOOD FOR: RECOVERY

BODYWEIGHT – LEGS

SIDE PLANK WITH HIP THRUST

▶ Lie on your side, elbow planted firmly on the floor directly below your shoulder. Bend your legs at a 90-degree angle, with your knees a little in front of your torso.

▶ Drive your bottom leg into the floor while you simultaneously lift your top leg. Your feet will separate; continue to drive your hips forward until fully extended, with the top leg up. The top of the position should look like a tall kneeling position in a side plank. In a controlled manner, return your legs and hips to the starting position. That's 1 rep.

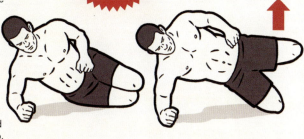

ALSO GOOD FOR:
BACK, ABS

SKATER LUNGE

▶ Start in an athletic stance, then lift your left foot off the floor. Leap to the left about 2 feet, landing only on your left foot; touch your right hand to the floor if needed. Jump off your left foot to the right, landing on your right foot. That's 1 rep. Repeat for prescribed number of reps.

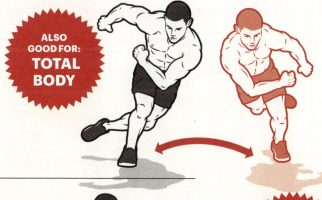

ALSO GOOD FOR:
TOTAL BODY

LATERAL LUNGE

▶ Stand with your feet wide apart, about double shoulder-width, with your toes pointing forward. Clasp your hands in front of your chest. This is the starting position. Shift your weight to your right foot and lower your body, pushing your hips back and bending your right knee until your right thigh is parallel to the floor. Return to the starting position and repeat to your left side. (Keep both feet on the floor throughout the move.) Continue alternating back and forth for the prescribed amount of time or reps.

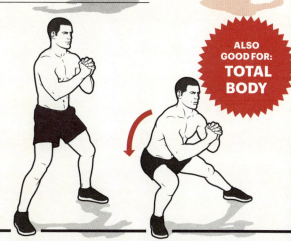

ALSO GOOD FOR:
TOTAL BODY

SPLIT SQUAT ISO HOLD

▶ Stand in a split squat position. Bend your knees to drop into a lunge; hold for the prescribed amount of time. Reverse and repeat on the other leg.

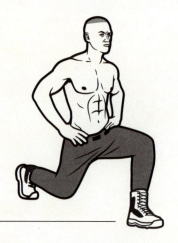

SPLIT SQUAT JUMP

▶ Assume a staggered stance with your right foot in front of your left. Lower your body into a lunge. Jump with enough force to propel both feet off the floor. Switch leg positions in the air so you land with your left leg forward. Alternate legs each rep. Continue for the prescribed amount of time.

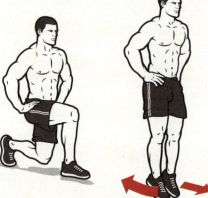

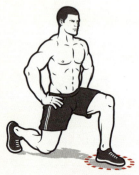

SUMO SQUAT STRETCH

▶ Stand with your feet shoulder-width apart. Go into a deep squat, keeping your chest up. When you're as deep as you feel comfortable, place your elbows on the insides of your knees. Hold for the prescribed amount of time.

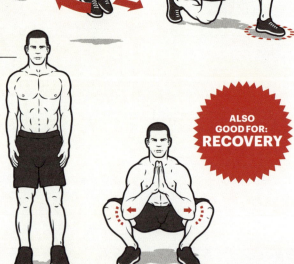

ALSO GOOD FOR: RECOVERY

BODYWEIGHT – TOTAL BODY

BURPEE

▶ Stand with your feet shoulder-width apart. Now push your hips back, lower your body as far as you can, and place your hands on the floor by your feet. Kick your legs back into a pushup position. Do a pushup (elbows tucked, body straight), and then bring your feet back to your hands and stand up. That's 1 rep. Perform for prescribed amount of time or number of reps.

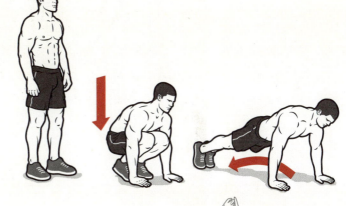

BROAD JUMP

▶ Stand a few inches behind a line. Leap forward as far as you can. Land on both feet with your knees bent. Turn around and jump back. Repeat for the prescribed amount of time.

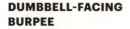

ALSO GOOD FOR: **LEGS**

DUMBBELL-FACING BURPEE

▶ Stand facing a pair of dumbbells placed on the floor in front of you. Do a burpee (see above); then hop over the dumbbells and turn to face them. That's 1 rep. Begin your next rep from there.

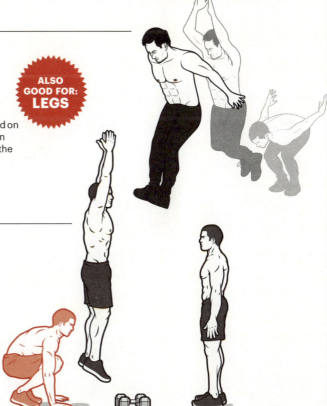

HIGH KNEE RUN

▶ Stand tall and run in place as fast as you can. Drive through the balls of your feet and try to bring your knees as high as possible. Your goal: Create a 90-degree angle in your knees. Keep your hands relaxed, elbows bent, and shoulders down, and swing your arms back and forth. Continue for the prescribed amount of time.

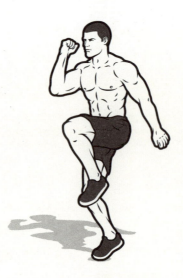

POWER SKIP

▶ Stand in an upright position with your hands at your sides. Slightly flex your left knee, then simultaneously and explosively push off the floor with your left leg and thrust your right knee toward the ceiling. Your right knee should be bent at a 90-degree angle, and your left arm should be bent into a running position (as if you were pumping your arm during a sprint). The goal is to jump vertically, not horizontally. Land on your left foot. Take a step forward with your right foot and, from a slightly flexed right knee, simultaneously push off the floor with your right foot and thrust your left knee. Continue for the prescribed amount of time.

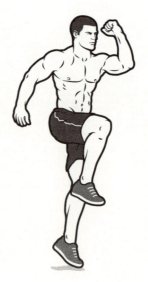
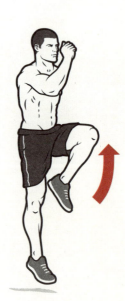

WEIGHTED – **ABS**

SINGLE RACK CARRY

▶ Stand upright, creating a strong, tall posture with abs and glutes engaged. Hold a kettlebell or dumbbell by your side. Lift the weight so it's high and tight against the upper part of your chest and your arm is tightly bent against your body.

▶ Walk forward, maintaining your tall posture and focusing on staying completely upright. Walk for the prescribed amount of time.

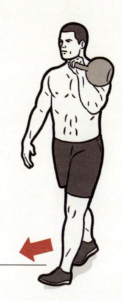

WEIGHTED – **ARMS**

DUMBBELL CURL

▶ Stand holding dumbbells at your sides, abs and glutes tight. Turn your arms so that your palms face forward.

▶ Keeping your upper arms next to your sides, bend your elbows and curl the dumbbells as close to your shoulders as you can. Pause, then slowly lower the weights back to the starting position. That's 1 rep. Each time you return to the starting position, completely straighten your arms. Repeat for the prescribed number of reps.

VARIATIONS

SPEED ALTERNATING DUMBBELL CURL

▶ Perform dumbbell curls as described but alternate arms at a brisk tempo. Each curl per arm equals 1 rep.

STANDING ALTERNATING DUMBBELL CURL

▶ Perform dumbbell curls as described but alternate arms. Each curl per arm is 1 rep. Each curl per each arm equals 1 rep.

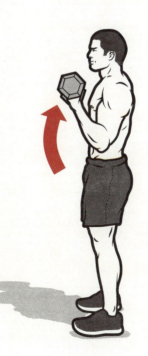

HAMMER CURL

▶ Stand upright, holding dumbbells at your sides, core tight. Keeping your entire body steady, curl the dumbbells upward with your palms facing each other, keeping your upper arms in the same position. Curl the weights until your elbows are bent slightly more than 90 degrees. Lower slowly to the starting position. That's 1 rep. Repeat for the prescribed number of reps.

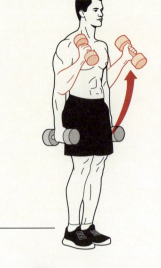

HINGE TO DUMBBELL TRICEPS KICKBACK

▶ Stand holding a pair of light dumbbells by your sides. Keeping your back straight and your legs slightly bent, hinge at the hips until your torso is almost parallel to the floor. Bend your elbows until your upper arms are parallel to the floor, keeping them close to your sides.

▶ Keeping your elbows and upper arms stationary, fully extend your forearms backward until your hands are slightly higher than your shoulders. Hold for a moment, squeezing your triceps hard.

▶ Bend your arms, lowering the weights, until your forearms are vertical. Stand and straighten your arms. That's 1 rep.

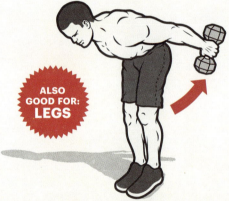

ALSO GOOD FOR: LEGS

LUNGE TO FRONT RAISE

▶ Stand tall, holding two light dumbbells by your sides. Take a big step forward with your left foot. Keeping your torso upright and both feet pointed forward, slowly bend both knees until your right knee is close to the floor.

▶ Holding the lunge position, slowly raise the dumbbells in front of you, keeping arms straight, until they reach shoulder height. Lower the dumbbells, step your left foot back to the starting position, and repeat the move with your right foot. That's 1 rep.

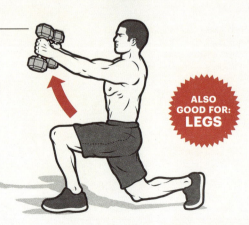

ALSO GOOD FOR: LEGS

WEIGHTED – ARMS

PLANK ALTERNATING ROW-TO-TRICEPS KICKBACK

▶ Holding a light dumbbell in each hand, get into a pushup position with your feet wider than shoulder width. Shift your weight onto your right hand. Bend your left elbow, keeping it close to your body, and raise the dumbbell in your left hand until your upper arm is parallel to the floor.

▶ Keeping your upper arm stationary, fully extend your forearm backward until your entire arm is parallel to the floor. Hold for a moment, then reverse the move, first bending your elbow until your forearm is vertical, then lowering the dumbbell back to the floor.

▶ Perform the same move with your opposite arm. That's 1 rep.

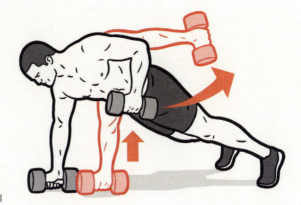

SEATED OVERHEAD DUMBBELL TRICEPS EXTENSION

▶ Grab a pair of dumbbells and sit on a bench or chair. Hold the dumbbells above your head, arms straight and your palms facing each other. Without moving your upper arms, lower the dumbbells behind your head. Pause, then straighten your arms to return the dumbbells to the starting overhead position. That's 1 rep. Repeat for the prescribed number of reps.

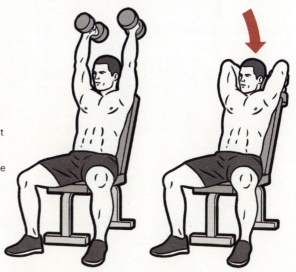

SIDE-LYING EXTERNAL ROTATION

▶ With a dumbbell in your right hand, lie on your left side; place a rolled towel under your right elbow if you want more support. Bend your left arm and rest your head on your left hand. Flex your right elbow to 90 degrees and rest the weight in front of your stomach. Don't bend your wrist. Keep your upper arm at your side as you rotate your right forearm to raise the weight until it's above your body. Slowly return to the starting position. That's 1 rep. Repeat for the prescribed number of reps.

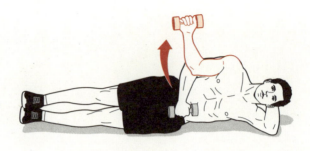

STANDING LATERAL RAISE

▶ Stand holding dumbbells at your sides, core and glutes tight, shoulder blades squeezed. Without bending your elbows, raise the weights out to your sides, elbows slightly in front of your torso, palms facing down. Pause when your elbows are nearly at shoulder height, then lower. That's 1 rep. Repeat for prescribed number of reps.

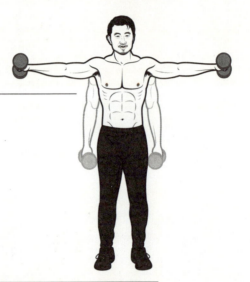

TALL KNEELING LATERAL DUMBBELL RAISE

▶ Holding a pair of dumbbells next to your sides, kneel on the floor with a tall posture, toes flexed and pressing into the floor.

▶ Keeping your core engaged and ribs down, and with a slight bend in your elbows, raise your arms straight out to your sides until they're at shoulder level. Pause for 1 second at the top of the movement, then slowly lower the weights back to the starting position at your sides. That's 1 rep. Perform for the prescribed amount of time.

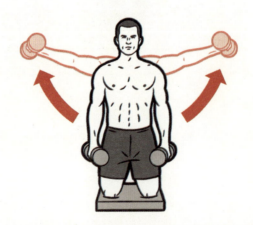

WEIGHTED — ARMS

TRICEPS KICKBACK

▶ Stand holding a pair of light dumbbells by your sides. Keeping your back straight and your legs slightly bent, hinge at the hips until your torso is almost parallel to the floor. Pull the dumbbells straight up until your elbows are against your sides. Keep them there throughout the movement. This is your starting position.

▶ Keeping your elbows stationary, fully extend your forearms backward until your arms are parallel to the floor. Hold for a moment, squeezing your triceps hard. Reverse the move and return to the starting position. That's 1 rep.

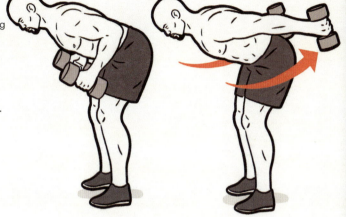

ZOTTMAN CURL

▶ Stand holding dumbbells at your sides, core and glutes tight. Without moving your upper arms and with your palms facing your torso, curl the weights toward your shoulders. At the top of the curl, rotate your wrists outward so your palms face forward. Keep them in this position and slowly lower the weights to the starting position. That's 1 rep. Repeat for the prescribed number of reps.

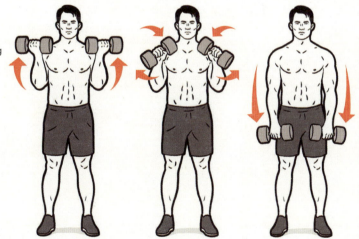

WEIGHTED – **BACK**

DEADLIFT TO ROW

▶ Stand holding dumbbells at your hips, abs and glutes tight, feet about shoulder-width apart. Keeping the dumbbells close to your legs, push your butt back and lower your torso until it's at a 45-degree angle with the floor. Tighten your abs. Now row the dumbbells to your ribcage, squeezing your shoulder blades. Reverse the moves back to the start.

FORM TIP: Row the weights up without moving your torso.

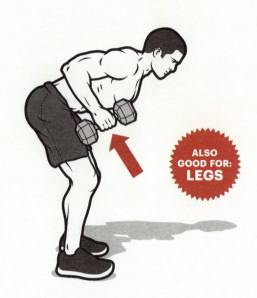

ALSO GOOD FOR: LEGS

SINGLE ARM DUMBBELL ROW

▶ Stand up straight, holding a dumbbell in your right hand. Bend your knees slightly, and hinge forward at your hips to lower your torso until it's almost parallel to the floor. Let the dumbbell hang from your shoulder. Pull the dumbbell up to the side of your torso, keeping your elbow tucked close to your side, then return it to start. That's 1 rep.

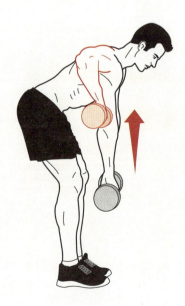

WEIGHTED – **BACK**

SINGLE LEG DEADLIFT TO ROW

▶ Stand tall, feet shoulder-width apart. Hold a medium-weight dumbbell in your left hand. Balance on your right foot and bend forward at the hips, extending your left leg behind you. Pull the dumbbell straight up to your ribs. Return to a standing position. That's 1 rep. Perform prescribed number of reps.

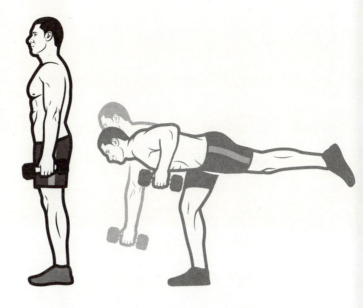

WEIGHTED – **CHEST**

CLOSE-GRIP FLOOR PRESS

▶ Lie faceup on the floor holding dumbbells above your chest, your arms straight and palms facing in. Lower the weights until your elbows touch the floor, keeping your upper arms close to your body. Press back up. That's 1 rep. Perform for prescribed amount of time.

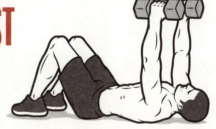

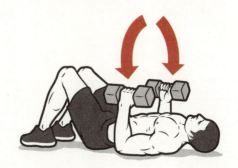

WEIGHTED – CHEST

FLOOR PRESS

▶ Lie on the floor, knees bent and feet flat. Hold dumbbells in both hands directly above your shoulders, core tight. Tighten your shoulder blades. This is the start. Bending at the shoulders and elbows, lower the dumbbells until your elbows touch the floor. Press back up, squeezing your chest. That's 1 rep. Repeat for the prescribed number of reps.

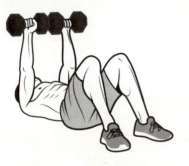

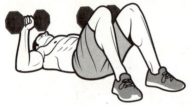

RENEGADE ROW

▶ Place a pair of dumbbells on the floor and grip them while you do a pushup. Once you're back in the starting position, row the dumbbell in your right hand up to the side of your chest. Lower the weight and repeat on your left side. That's 1 rep. Perform prescribed number of reps.

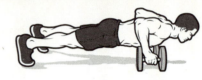

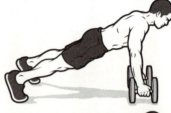

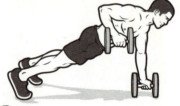

WEIGHTED – LEGS

ALTERNATING OVERHEAD REVERSE LUNGE

▶ Hold a pair of dumbbells overhead, arms extended straight up, your feet shoulder-width apart. Step back with your right leg into a lunge, pause, and return to the starting position. Repeat on the left side. That's 1 rep.

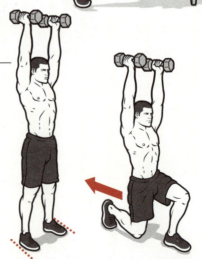

WEIGHTED — LEGS

DOUBLE KETTLEBELL SWING

▶ Place two kettlebells or dumbbells on the floor in front of you. Stand with your feet slightly wider than your shoulders, push your hips back, and grab the weights. Pull the weights up, "hike" them back between your legs, then thrust your hips forward as you swing both weights up to chest level. Swing the weights back between your legs. That's 1 rep; continue without pausing.

ALSO GOOD FOR: **BACK, TOTAL BODY**

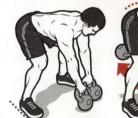
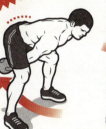
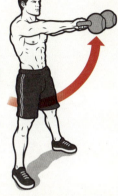

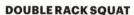

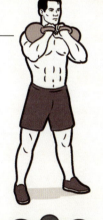
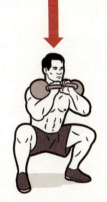

DOUBLE RACK SQUAT

▶ Stand holding kettlebells at your shoulders, elbows tucked, glutes and abs tight. Push your butt back slightly and bend your knees, lowering your torso until your thighs are parallel with the floor. Stand back up. That's 1 rep.

DUMBBELL FRONT SQUAT

▶ Stand upright, feet shoulder-width apart, holding a dumbbell at each shoulder. Making sure your knees don't extend past your toes, squat slowly, taking 3 seconds to descend until your hips are below your knees. Explode back to a standing position. That's 1 rep. Repeat for prescribed amount of time.

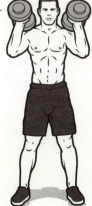
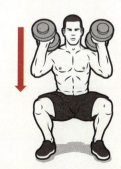

ALSO GOOD FOR: **TOTAL BODY**

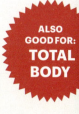

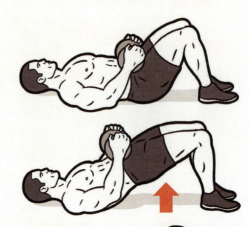

DUMBBELL GLUTE BRIDGE

▶ Lie faceup on the floor with your knees bent and your heels on the floor. Hold a dumbbell at your hip bones.

▶ Driving your heels into the floor, raise your hips so your body forms a straight line from your shoulders to your knees. Hold this position for the prescribed amount of time.

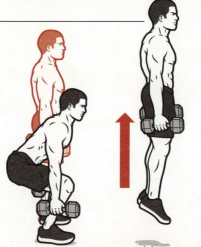

DUMBBELL JUMP SQUAT

▶ Stand with your feet shoulder-width apart, holding a pair of dumbbells at your sides. Pushing your hips back and bending your knees, lower your torso as far as you can. Pause, then straighten your legs and explosively jump up. Land as softly as possible. That's 1 rep. Repeat for prescribed number of reps.

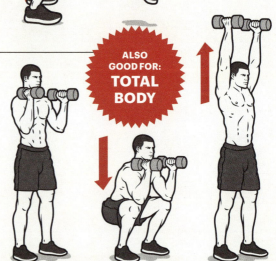

ALSO GOOD FOR: TOTAL BODY

DUMBBELL SQUAT PRESS

▶ Stand with feet about shoulder-width apart, holding a pair of dumbbells in front of your shoulders. Keep your abs and glutes engaged. Squat as deeply as you can, then explode up. As you rise, thrust the weights straight above your shoulders. Return to the starting position. That's 1 rep. Continue for the prescribed amount of time.

WEIGHTED – LEGS

DUMBBELL SWING

▶ With feet shoulder-width apart, hold a dumbbell handle with both hands. Bend at the waist, bend your knees slightly, push your hips back, and lower your torso. Swing the dumbbell between your legs, then thrust your hips forward and swing the weight up to shoulder height, arms extended. Immediately swing the weight back between your legs. Keep swinging for the prescribed number of reps.

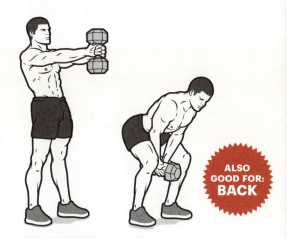

ALSO GOOD FOR: BACK

GOBLET ALTERNATING REVERSE LUNGE

▶ Stand tall and hold a hold a kettlebell or dumbbell at your chest with both hands, core tight. Step back with your right leg, lowering into a lunge until your left thigh is parallel to the floor. Explosively stand back up. Repeat on the other side. That's 1 rep. Repeat for prescribed number of reps.

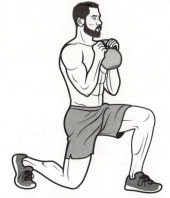

SINGLE- LEG ROMANIAN DEADLIFT

▶ Stand holding a dumbbell in your left hand at your hips, core tight. Lift your left foot off the floor, then, keeping your hips and shoulders square, hinge forward. Lower until your torso is nearly parallel to the floor or you can't keep your balance, whichever comes first. Keep your left leg in line with your torso as you do this. Return to standing, squeezing your glutes. That's 1 rep. Repeat for prescribed number of reps.

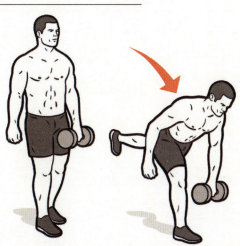

WEIGHTED – **TOTAL BODY**

ALTERNATING DUMBBELL SNATCH

▶ Stand explosively (you may elevate onto your toes as you do) and squeeze your glutes. Pull the weight upward as you do this, keeping it close to your torso the entire time. As it reaches shoulder height, pull it close to your body, then punch toward the ceiling. Lower to your shoulder, then lower to the start. That's 1 rep; repeat for the prescribed number of reps.

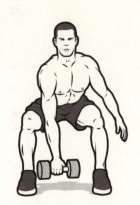
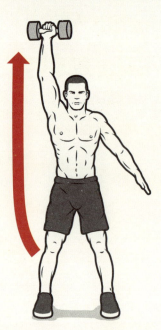

ALTERNATING TURKISH GETUP

▶ Lie on your back on the floor, legs straight, and hold a hold a kettlebell or dumbbell overhead in your right hand. Stand up while keeping the weight overhead at all times. Return to the starting position and repeat with the weight in your left hand. That's 1 rep. Repeat for the prescribed amount of time.

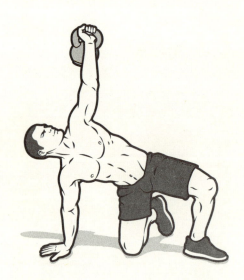

RECOVERY

3-LEGGED DOG

▶ Start in a plank position. Push your tailbone toward your heels, extend your chest, and brace your core. Your upper arms should wrap outward to broaden your chest. Inhale, lift your hips, and push your butt up into the air. Draw in your rib cage and press your legs back. Extend your heels away from your toes and push them into the floor. Lift your left leg, keeping your hips square to the floor. Hold for the prescribed amount of time then bring your left foot back to the floor. Repeat on the right side.

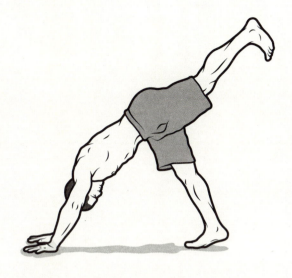

ARM JOINT CIRCLE

▶ Hold arms straight out to your sides, palms forward. Start with small circles and progress to larger ones. Continue for the prescribed amount of time.

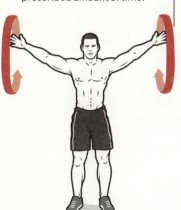

HIP JOINT CIRCLE

▶ Place your hands on your hips, guiding them through exaggerated circles. Continue for the prescribed amount of time.

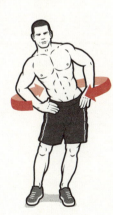

KNEE JOINT CIRCLE

▶ Place your feet together so that your knees touch. Now bend your knees and place your hands on them, guiding them through exaggerated circles. Continue for the prescribed amount of time.

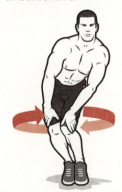

COBRA STRETCH

▶ Lie flat on your stomach, hands next to your shoulders and the tops of your feet on the floor.

▶ Using your hands, gently push your upper body up until you have extended as far as you're comfortable. Let your belly relax and your lower back tense as you prop yourself on your hands (or forearms if you can't make it to a straight-arm position). Hold, relax, and breathe for the prescribed amount of time. Return to starting position.

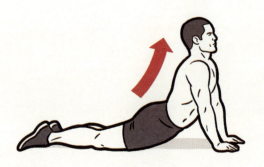

LUNGE STRETCH

▶ From standing, step one foot forward, then bend your front knee. Hold for the prescribed amount of time. Return to starting position.

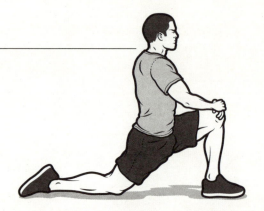

PRONE SHOULDER IR/ER

▶ Lie flat on your stomach with both arms extended. Begin with your right palm facing up toward the ceiling and your left palm facing down toward the floor. While maintaining a stable rib position, flip your hands to the opposite side with the palm-down hand changing to palm up and vice versa. Once both hands have switched positions, switch them back to their original position. That's 1 rep. Repeat for prescribed amount of time.

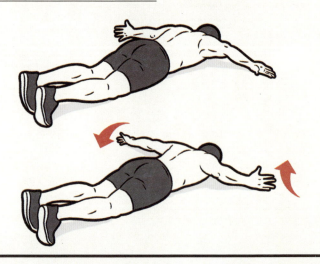

RECOVERY

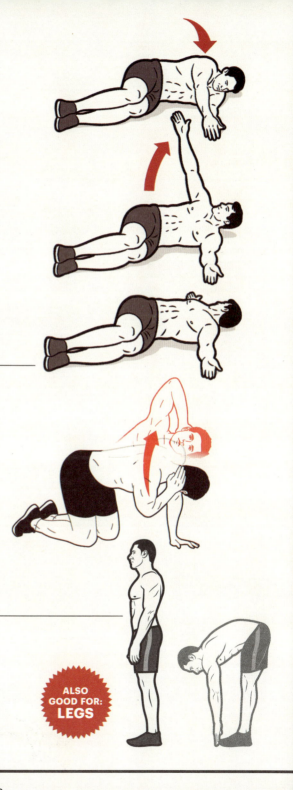

SIDE-LYING T-SPINE ROTATION

▶ Begin by lying on your left side with knees bent 90 degrees and arms straight out in front of you, palms touching.

▶ Gently lift your right hand straight up off your left hand, opening up the arm like it's a book or door while following the top hand with your head and eyes until your right hand is on the other side of your body, palm up, with your head and eyes turned toward the right. Hold this stretch for a few breaths before returning to the starting position with palms facing each other. Continue rolling over for the prescribed amount of time.

THORACIC ROTATION

▶ Position yourself on the floor on your hands and knees, hands below shoulders and knees below hips. Place your right hand behind your head so your elbow points out to the side. Brace your core and rotate your right shoulder toward your left arm, pointing your right elbow toward the floor. Follow your elbow with your eyes as you reverse the movement until your right elbow points toward the ceiling. That's 1 rep. Perform the prescribed number of reps, then switch arms and repeat on the other side.

TOE TOUCH

▶ Stand with your feet together, knees locked. Hinge forward and reach for the floor. Your goal is to touch the floor with your fingertips or, at the very least, be just 2 inches short of that goal. Hold for the prescribed amount of time.

ALSO GOOD FOR: LEGS

SUPINE LEG SWITCH

▶ Lie on the floor with your legs extended and arms at 45-degree angles away from your body. Lift your legs 6 inches off the floor by engaging your core and hip flexors.

▶ Shift your right leg up and left leg down, then cross them over each other. Reverse the pattern, and shift your right leg under your left leg, crossing them over each other. When you return back to both feet together, that's 1 rep. Continue for the prescribed amount of time.

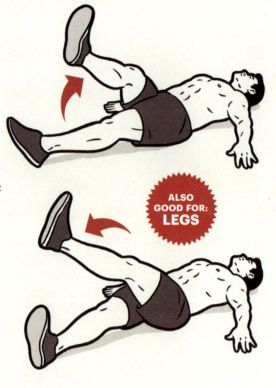

ALSO GOOD FOR: LEGS

WORLD'S GREATEST STRETCH

▶ Get into the pushup position, keeping your back straight and squeezing your glutes and core.

▶ Drive your left leg forward as if you were Spider-Man. Plant your full foot to create strong contact with the floor. Once stable, lift your left hand off the floor and turn your upper body so that your hand reaches directly toward the ceiling as you straighten your arm. Keep your eyes on your hand while turning your body. Slowly rotate your body so your hand returns to the floor and your foot returns to the pushup position. Repeat this move on the right side; that's 1 rep.

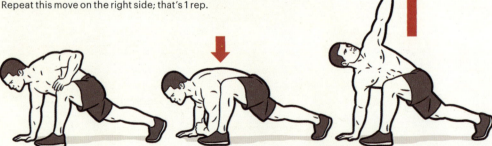

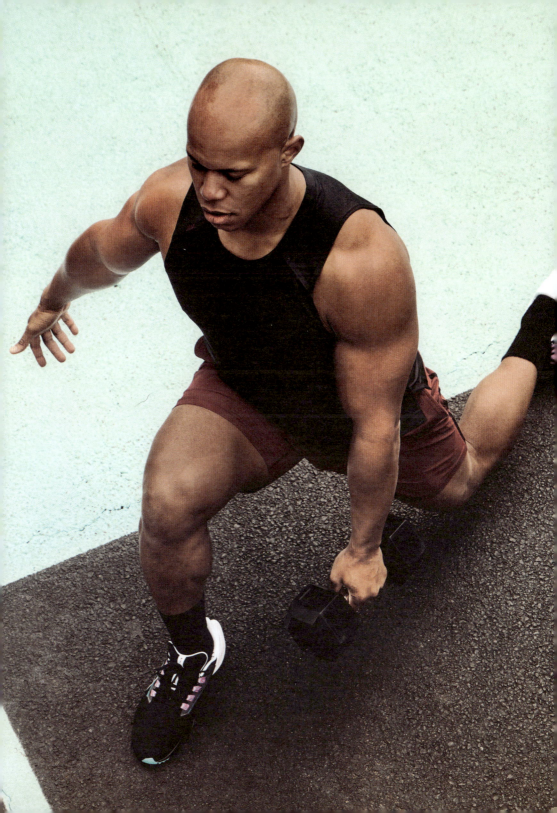

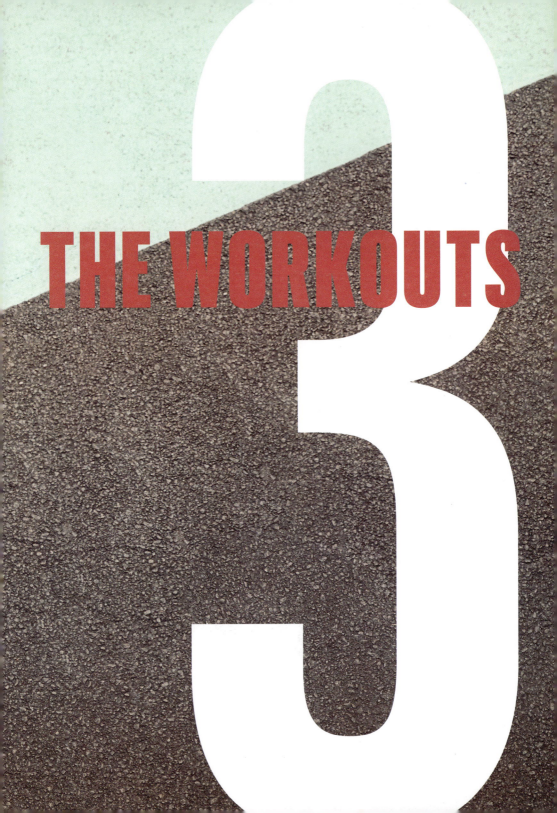

THE WORKOUTS

3

MEET YOUR
TRAINERS

We tapped some of the fittest (and most time-strapped) experts we know to share their best seven-minute workouts.

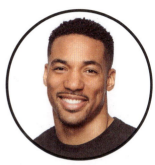

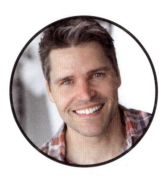

DAVID FREEMAN

Here to provide your dose of weighted back, bodyweight ab, and total body workouts is David Freeman, NASM. He's the National Digital Performer Brand Leader at Life Time Fitness and the creator of the Freeman Method, a kettlebell-focused program on All Out Studio. He's trained several NFL players. He played professional football overseas before finding his calling as a fitness professional.

DAVID'S WORKOUTS
Bodyweight Abs (p. 86), Weighted Back (p. 110), Bodyweight Total Body (p. 76)

ANDREW HEFFERNAN

Andrew Heffernan, CSCS, is a fitness coach, a Feldenkrais practitioner, and your guide through the first section of this book. For almost 20 years, he has developed safe and effective fitness solutions for actors, older clients, and athletes alike, and he built all the arm and weighted ab workouts you'll find in the coming pages.

ANDREW'S WORKOUTS
Weighted Abs (p. 90), Bodyweight Arms (p. 96), Weighted Arms (p. 100)

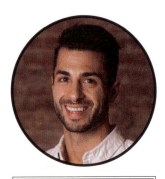

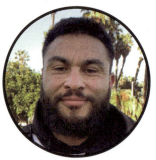

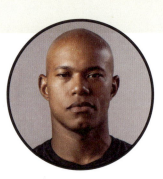

DANIEL GIORDANO

As a cofounder of Bespoke Treatments, a physical-therapy clinic in New York City that specializes in sports and orthopedic rehab, Daniel Giordano, PT, DPT, CSCS, is exactly who you want building your recovery workouts (which is why we had him create them for us). He also developed the bodyweight back workouts in this book. Giordano is a Men's Health advisor and the creator of the Daily Mobility workout program on All Out Studio.

DANIEL'S WORKOUTS
Recovery (p. 136),
Bodyweight Back (p. 106)

JUAN GUADARRAMA

What do you get when you combine the agility of an elite soccer player with the muscle and power of a strength coach? Competitive powerlifter and owner of California gym Sorta HQ, Juan Guadarrama. After leaving the soccer field, Guadarrama pivoted to coaching functional fitness and powerlifting. Here he serves up a few fat-burning leg and weighted total-body sessions.

JUAN'S WORKOUTS
Weighted Legs (p. 130),
Bodyweight Legs (p. 126),
Weighted Total Body
(p. 80)

JAHKEEN WASHINGTON

The mind behind all the chest workouts in this book is Jahkeen Washington, Men's Health 2020 Top Trainer winner and founder of JTW FIT and Harlem Kettlebell Club in NYC. Washington coaches clients using various modalities, though all you'll need to crush the workouts here is a set of dumbbells and seven minutes. His motto: "if you don't work, nothing works."

JAHKEEN'S WORKOUTS
Bodyweight Chest (p. 116),
Weighted Chest (p. 120)

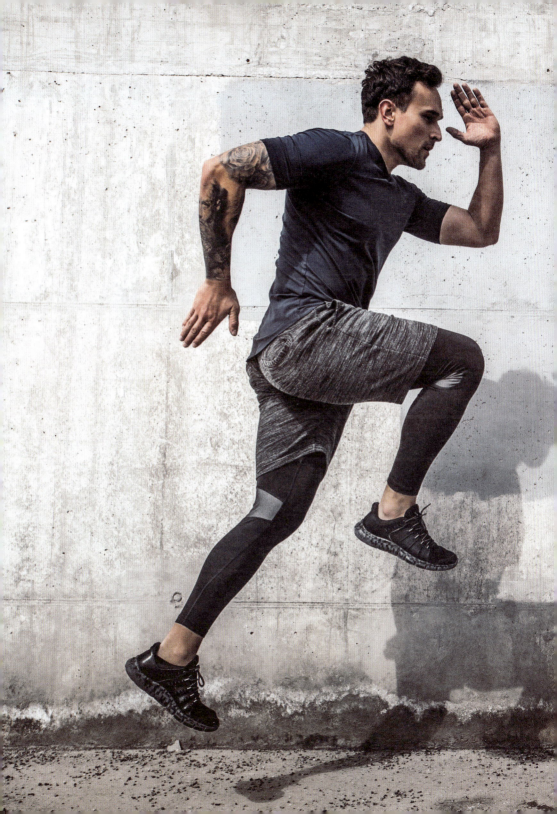

SEVEN-MINUTE
TOTAL–BODY
WORKOUTS

IN THE 1950S and '60s, even the most dedicated physique athletes trained their entire body each time they worked out. Buzzing through exercises for their arms, legs, abs, and entire trunk, with minimal rest between moves, they built lean, muscular physiques that impress to this day. Their old-school approach can work for you, too—even in seven minutes. As you transition quickly from floor moves to standing moves and back again, working the body as a single unit, you'll build not just strength and muscle but also coordination, athleticism, and cardiovascular endurance: that's both show and go, together in one fast, efficient package.

IF YOU HAVE MORE THAN SEVEN MINUTES...

Before each of these workouts, get your body primed quickly by doing 30 seconds each of jumping jacks and reverse lunges, followed by a reverse plank. Then jump into the action.

BODYWEIGHT – **TOTAL BODY**

THE FULL-BODY EXPLOSIVE CRUSHER

CIRCUIT 1	WORK	REST
REVERSE LUNGE (R)	40 sec.	20 sec.
REVERSE LUNGE (L)	40 sec.	20 sec.
BURPEE	40 sec.	20 sec.
Complete 2 rounds of this circuit.		

FINISHER	WORK	REST
BROAD JUMP	60 sec.	None

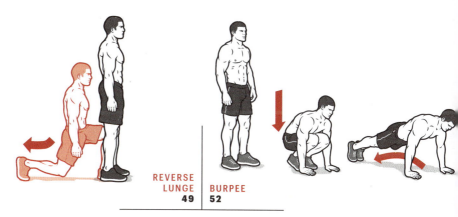

REVERSE LUNGE
49

BURPEE
52

52
BROAD JUMP

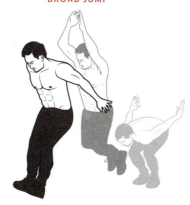

BODYWEIGHT – **TOTAL BODY**

HIGH-REP MUSCLE MAYHEM

6-MIN. EMOM	WORK ·	REST
REVERSE LUNGE	20 reps	This is an EMOM workout. Begin each move at the start of a minute. Complete the reps, then use the remaining time in the minute as your rest.
SKATER LUNGE	20 reps	
BODYWEIGHT SQUAT	15 reps	
Complete 2 rounds of this circuit.		

FINISHER	WORK	REST
PLYO PUSHUP	60 sec.	None

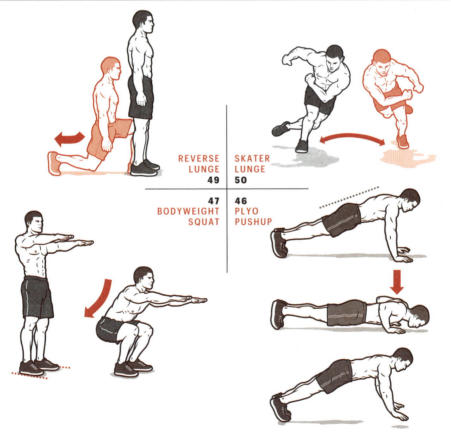

REVERSE LUNGE
49

SKATER LUNGE
50

47
BODYWEIGHT SQUAT

46
PLYO PUSHUP

BODYWEIGHT – **TOTAL BODY**

PLANK-POSITION FULL-BODY BLAST

CIRCUIT 1	WORK	REST
PLANK JACK	30 sec.	15 sec.
JUMP SQUAT	30 sec.	15 sec.
PUSHUP	30 sec.	15 sec.
Complete 2 rounds of this circuit.		

FINISHER	WORK	REST
PLANK WITH KNEE TO ELBOW	60 sec.	None

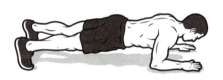

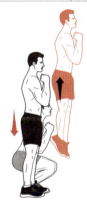

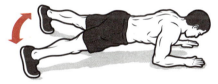

PLANK JACK
36

JUMP SQUAT
49

46
PUSHUP

37
PLANK WITH KNEE TO ELBOW

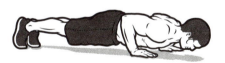

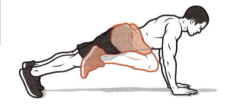

BODYWEIGHT – TOTAL BODY

METABOLIC INTERVAL MADNESS

CIRCUIT 1	WORK	REST
HIGH KNEE RUN	30 sec.	30 sec.
BEAST TAP	30 sec.	30 sec.
SPLIT SQUAT JUMP	30 sec.	30 sec.
Complete 2 rounds of this circuit.		

FINISHER	WORK	REST
POWER SKIP	60 sec.	None

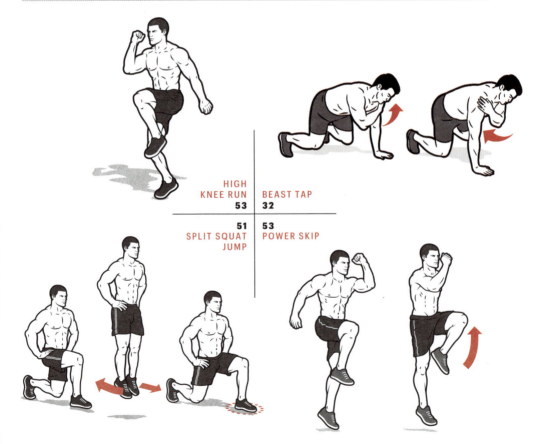

HIGH KNEE RUN
53

BEAST TAP
32

51
SPLIT SQUAT JUMP

53
POWER SKIP

WEIGHTED – **TOTAL BODY**

ULTIMATE UPPER-BODY MUSCLE

SUPERSET	WORK	REST
STANDING LATERAL RAISE	20 reps	None
SINGLE ARM DUMBBELL ROW (R)	20 reps	None
SINGLE ARM DUMBBELL ROW (L)	20 reps	None
Complete 2 rounds of this superset. Rest 60 sec. between rounds.		

3-MIN. AMRAP	WORK	REST
ALTERNATING TURKISH GETUP	AMRAP in 3 min.	Rest as needed, but aim to keep moving for 3 full min.

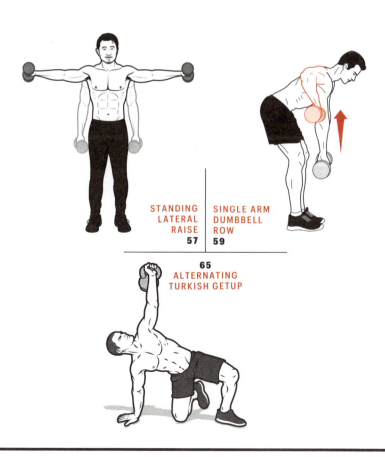

STANDING LATERAL RAISE
57

SINGLE ARM DUMBBELL ROW
59

65
ALTERNATING TURKISH GETUP

WEIGHTED – **TOTAL BODY**

HIGH-REP STRENGTH AND EXPLOSIVENESS

SUPERSET	WORK	REST
SEATED OVERHEAD DUMBBELL TRICEPS EXTENSION	20 reps	None
FLOOR PRESS	20 reps	None
Complete 2 rounds of this superset. Rest 60 sec. between rounds.		
ALTERNATING DUMBBELL SNATCH	60 reps	None

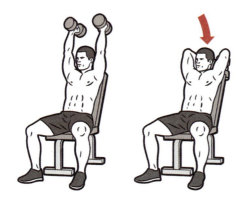

SEATED OVERHEAD DUMBBELL
TRICEP EXTENSION
56

61
FLOOR
PRESS

65
ALTERNATING
DUMBBELL
SNATCH

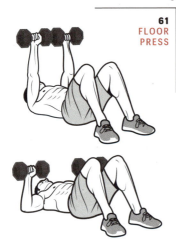

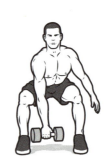

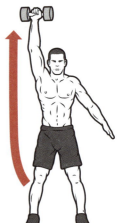

WEIGHTED – **TOTAL BODY**

THE SQUAT-TO-PRESS CRUSHER

7-MIN. EMOM	WORK	REST
DUMBBELL SQUAT PRESS	15 reps	This is an EMOM series. Begin a set of squat presses at the start of a minute. Complete the reps, then use the remaining time in the minute as your rest.

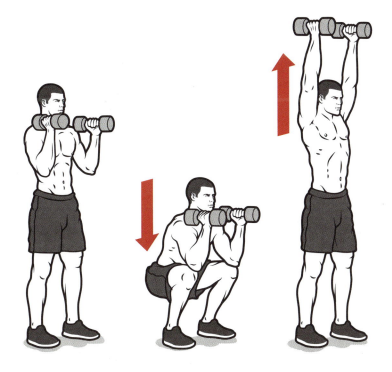

63
DUMBBELL SQUAT PRESS

WEIGHTED – **TOTAL BODY**

THE CARRY-AND-LUNGE BLAST

SUPERSET	WORK	REST
SINGLE RACK CARRY (R)	30 sec.	None
SINGLE RACK CARRY (L)	30 sec.	None
SIDE-LYING EXTERNAL ROTATION (R)	30 sec.	None
SIDE-LYING EXTERNAL ROTATION (L)	30 sec.	None
ALTERNATING OVERHEAD REVERSE LUNGE	60 sec.	None
Complete 2 rounds of this superset. Rest 30 sec. between rounds.		

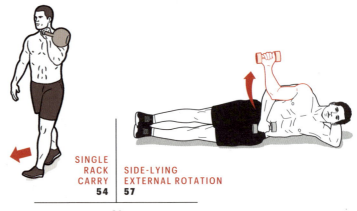

SINGLE RACK CARRY
54

SIDE-LYING EXTERNAL ROTATION
57

61
ALTERNATING OVERHEAD REVERSE LUNGE

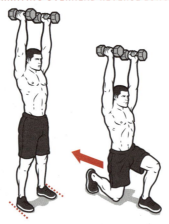

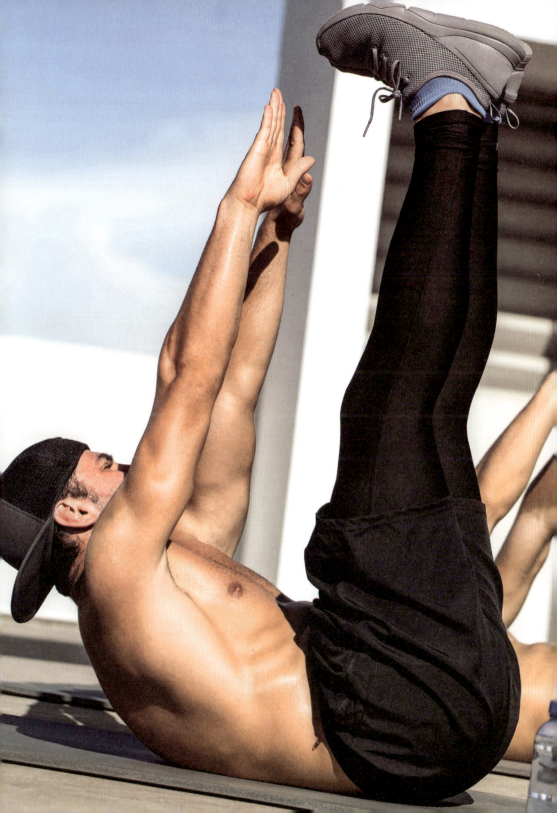

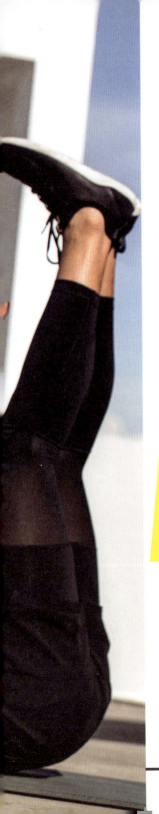

SEVEN-MINUTE
AB
WORKOUTS

ABS ARE HIGH on everyone's list of muscles they'd like to develop. They keep your back healthy and pain-free, they improve your posture, and they look great in board shorts. The big mistake many people make in pursuit of the coveted six-pack, however, is to work their ab muscles too much and too hard, leading to listless, ineffective workouts and stalled progress. In truth, seven minutes is plenty of time to get a solid workout in for your entire waist, including the rectus abdominis (six-pack muscle), the internal and external obliques (on the sides of your waist), and the intercostals (between the ribs on the sides of your rib cage). Together, these muscles rotate, bend, flex, and extend your torso in all directions, making them essential players in athletics and everyday life. Like your legs, the abs are used to hard work, so don't hold back in these workouts— your six-pack awaits.

THE ALL-AROUND CORE CRUSHER

CIRCUIT 1	WORK	REST
BEAR CRAWL	40 sec.	20 sec.
V-UP	40 sec.	20 sec.
BODYWEIGHT WIPER	40 sec.	20 sec.
Complete 2 rounds of this circuit.		

FINISHER	WORK	REST
BICYCLE CRUNCH	60 sec.	None

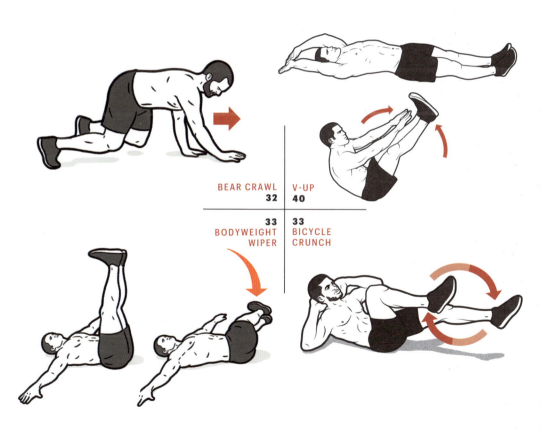

BEAR CRAWL
32

V-UP
40

33
BODYWEIGHT
WIPER

33
BICYCLE
CRUNCH

BODYWEIGHT – ABS

THE ABDOMINAL AND LOWER-BACK BLAST

CIRCUIT 1	WORK	REST
PLANK	30 sec.	30 sec.
DEADBUG	30 sec.	30 sec.
SUPERMAN	30 sec.	30 sec.
Complete 2 rounds of this circuit.		

FINISHER	WORK	REST
PLANK WITH KNEE TO ELBOW	60 sec.	None

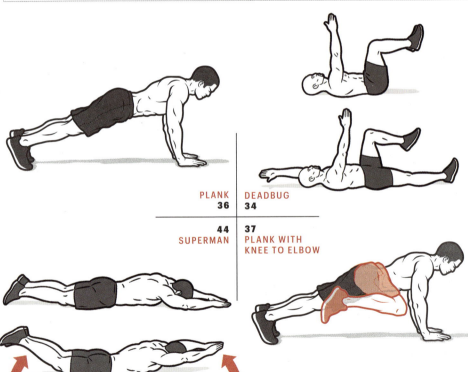

PLANK
36

DEADBUG
34

44
SUPERMAN

37
PLANK WITH
KNEE TO ELBOW

BODYWEIGHT – ABS

THE FUNCTIONAL CORE CRUSHER

CIRCUIT 1	WORK	REST
REVERSE CRUNCH	25 reps	This is an EMOM (every minute on the minute) workout. Begin each move at the start of a minute. Complete the reps, then use the remaining time in the minute as your rest.
SHOULDER TAP (FROM PUSHUP POSITION)	20 reps	
SUPINE LEG LIFT	15 reps	
Complete 2 rounds of this circuit.		

FINISHER	SETS	WORK	REST
CRAB GRAB	2	25 reps	None

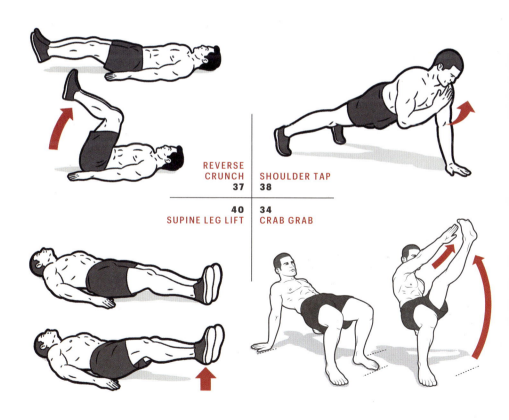

REVERSE CRUNCH
37

SHOULDER TAP
38

40
SUPINE LEG LIFT

34
CRAB GRAB

BODYWEIGHT – ABS

THE HOLDS-FOCUSED CORE CRUSHER

CIRCUIT 1	WORK	REST
SUPINE LEG SWITCH	20 sec.	10 sec.
HOLLOW HOLD	20 sec.	10 sec.
BEAR REVERSE CRAWL	20 sec.	10 sec.
Complete 4 rounds of this circuit.		

FINISHER	WORK	REST
BEAR CRAWL	30 sec.	None

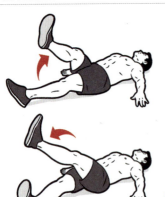

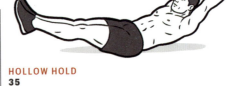

SUPINE
LEG
SWITCH
69

HOLLOW HOLD
35

32
BEAR
REVERSE
CRAWL

32
BEAR CRAWL

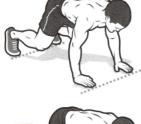

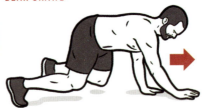

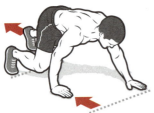

WEIGHTED – ABS

THE WEIGHTED BASICS ROUTINE

CIRCUIT 1	WORK	REST
V-UP WITH WEIGHTS	45 sec.	15 sec.
SUPERMAN WITH WEIGHTS	45 sec.	15 sec.
SIDE PLANK	30 sec. per side	60 sec.
Complete 2 rounds of this circuit.		

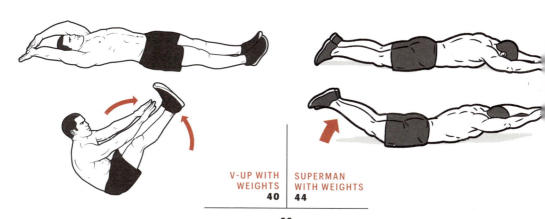

V-UP WITH
WEIGHTS
40

SUPERMAN
WITH WEIGHTS
44

38
SIDE PLANK

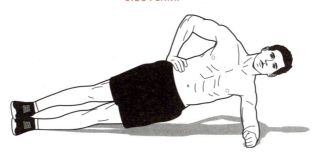

WEIGHTED – ABS

CORE BASICS AND CARRIES

CIRCUIT 1	WORK	REST
HOLLOW BODY CRUNCH ROCK	12 reps	None
PLANK WITH LEG LIFT	15 reps	None
HOLLOW HOLD	45 sec.	None
SINGLE RACK CARRY (R)	25 steps	None
SINGLE RACK CARRY (L)	25 steps	None
Complete 2 rounds of this circuit. Rest 30 sec. between rounds.		

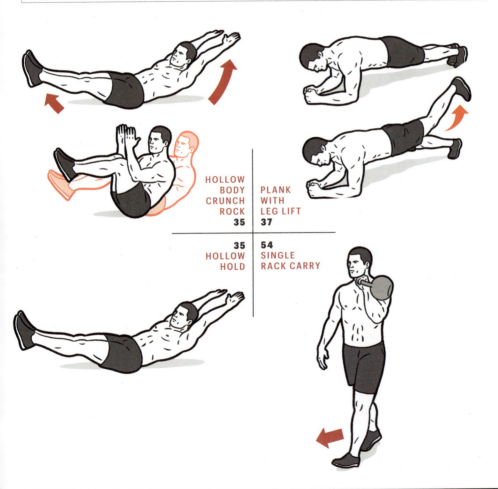

HOLLOW BODY CRUNCH ROCK
35

PLANK WITH LEG LIFT
37

35
HOLLOW HOLD

54
SINGLE RACK CARRY

WEIGHTED – ABS

THE ULTIMATE AB CHIPPER

CIRCUIT 1	WORK	REST
SIDE PLANK OVER AND BACK (R)	12 reps	As little as possible
SIDE PLANK OVER AND BACK (L)	12 reps	As little as possible
CRAB GRAB	12 reps	As little as possible
SIDE PLANK WITH TOP ARM REACH (R)	12 reps	As little as possible
SIDE PLANK WITH TOP ARM REACH (L)	12 reps	As little as possible
DEADBUG (LIGHT DUMBBELLS) (R)	12 reps	As little as possible
DEADBUG (LIGHT DUMBBELLS) (L)	12 reps	As little as possible
SIDE PLANK (R)	30 sec.	As little as possible
SIDE PLANK (L)	30 sec.	As little as possible
LYING DUMBBELL LEG LIFT	15 reps	As little as possible

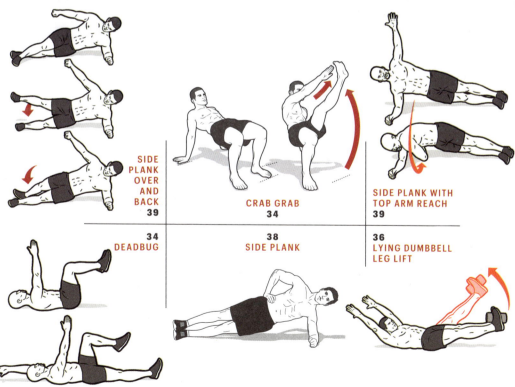

SIDE PLANK OVER AND BACK
39

CRAB GRAB
34

SIDE PLANK WITH TOP ARM REACH
39

34
DEADBUG

38
SIDE PLANK

36
LYING DUMBBELL LEG LIFT

WEIGHTED – ABS

THE HEAVYWEIGHT CORE BLAST

CIRCUIT 1	WORK	REST
PLANK JACK	25 reps	None
SINGLE RACK CARRY (R)	40 reps	None
SINGLE RACK CARRY (L)	40 reps	None
WEIGHTED HOLLOW HOLD (LIGHT WEIGHTS)	30 reps	None
Complete 3 rounds of this circuit. Rest 30 sec. between rounds.		

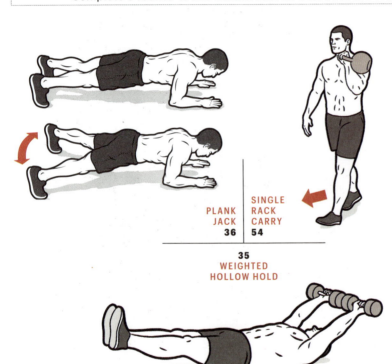

PLANK JACK
36

SINGLE RACK CARRY
54

35
WEIGHTED HOLLOW HOLD

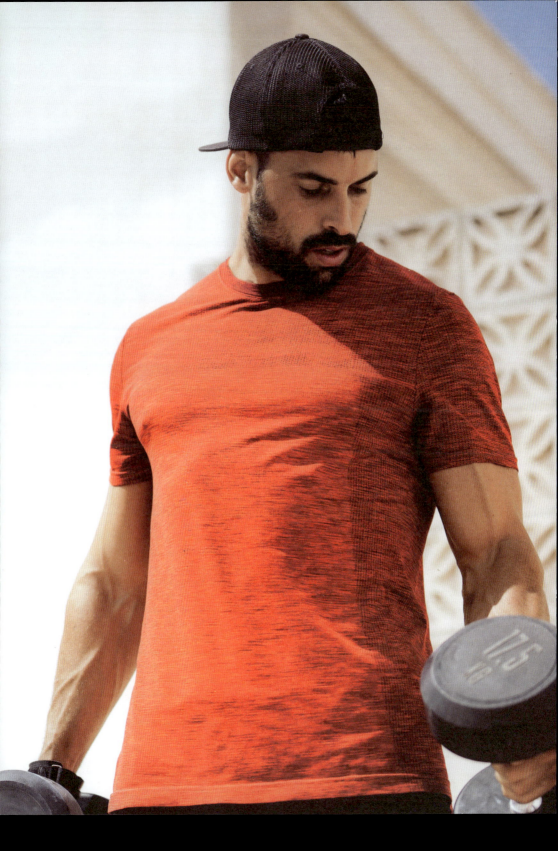

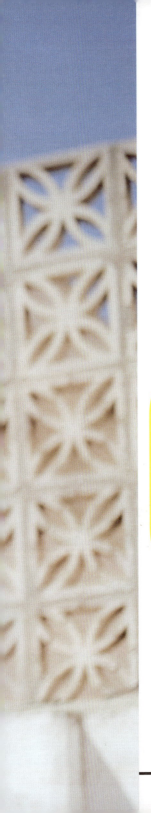

SEVEN-MINUTE
ARM
WORKOUTS

COMPARED TO THE slabs of sinew on your legs and torso, your arm muscles are relatively small. That's good news for you and your crammed schedule. The biceps (which flex your elbow), the triceps (which extend it), and the many muscles of the forearms (which flex and extend your wrists and fingers) don't demand a lot of oxygen when they work, which means you can blaze through seven minutes of arm work with relatively little rest, catching a Herculean pump while stimulating new strength and muscle in record time. Arm sessions are tough, but they don't take a lot out of you—making them among the most fun workouts in this book.

BODYWEIGHT – ARMS

THE REPS-AND-HOLDS TRICEPS CRUSHER

CIRCUIT 1	WORK	REST
FRENCH PRESS PUSHUP	8 reps	None
ISO TRICEPS SQUEEZE	8 reps	None
CLOSE-GRIP PUSHUP	8 reps	None
ISO TRICEPS SQUEEZE	8 reps	None
PUSHUP	8 reps	None
ISO TRICEPS SQUEEZE	8 reps	None
HANDS-ELEVATED CLOSE-GRIP PUSHUP	8 reps	None
ISO TRICEPS SQUEEZE	8 reps	None
Repeat this circuit for as many rounds as possible (AMRAP).		

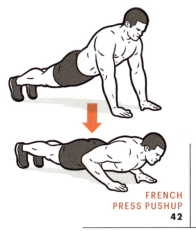

FRENCH
PRESS PUSHUP
42

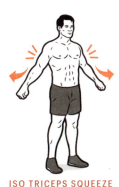
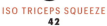

ISO TRICEPS SQUEEZE
42

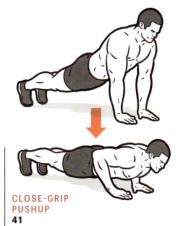

CLOSE-GRIP
PUSHUP
41

46
PUSHUP

41
HANDS-ELEVATED
CLOSE-GRIP
PUSHUP

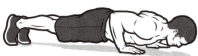

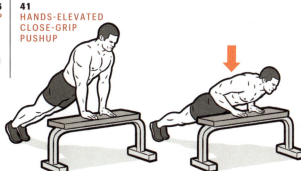

BODYWEIGHT – ARMS

THE TRIS AND REAR-DELTS BLAST

CIRCUIT 1	WORK	REST
CLOSE-GRIP PUSHUP	1 rep	None
REVERSE T-RAISE	1 rep	None
Complete 10 rounds of this circuit, increasing reps by 1 each round. Rest 10 sec. between rounds.		

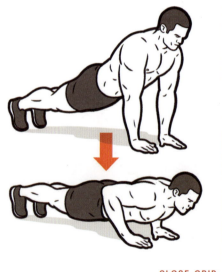

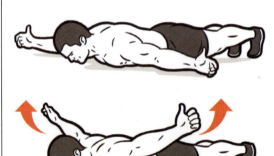

CLOSE-GRIP
PUSHUP
41

REVERSE
T-RAISE
44

BODYWEIGHT – ARMS

ENDURANCE TRICEPS AND SHOULDERS

CIRCUIT 1	WORK	REST
FRENCH PRESS PUSHUP	5 reps	None
CLOSE-GRIP T-STOP PUSHUP	Stop 3 reps shy of failure	None
BEAR CRAWL	20 steps per side	None
Complete 4 rounds of this circuit. Rest 1 min. between rounds. Perform Close-Grip T-Stop Pushup to failure on your final round.		

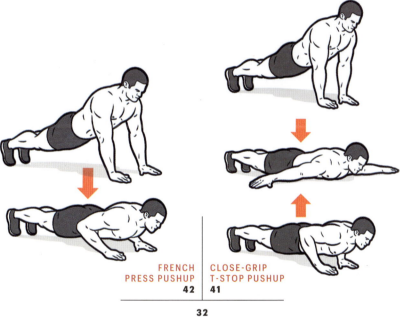

FRENCH
PRESS PUSHUP
42

CLOSE-GRIP
T-STOP PUSHUP
41

32
BEAR CRAWL

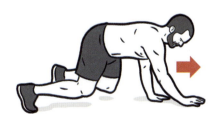

BODYWEIGHT – ARMS

THE PUSHUP SUPERSETS SESSION

CIRCUIT 1	WORK	REST
FRENCH PRESS PUSHUP	4 reps	None
HANDS-ELEVATED PUSHUP	6 reps	None
Repeat this circuit as many times as possible in 3 min. Rest and stretch 1 min.		
CIRCUIT 2	WORK	REST
BEAR CRAWL	10 steps	None
HANDS-ELEVATED PUSHUP	6 reps	None
Repeat this circuit as many times as possible in 3 min.		

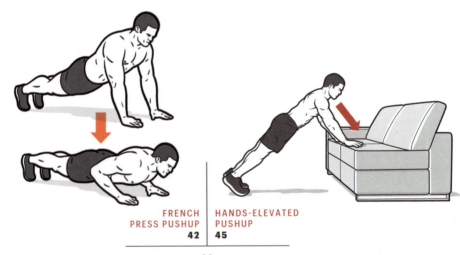

FRENCH PRESS PUSHUP
42

HANDS-ELEVATED PUSHUP
45

32
BEAR CRAWL

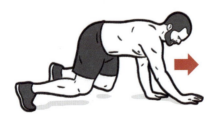

WEIGHTED – ARMS

BACK-AND-FORTH BICEPS AND TRICEPS

CIRCUIT 1	WORK	REST
SEATED OVERHEAD DUMBBELL TRICEPS EXTENSION	12 reps	None
HAMMER CURL	12 reps	None
TRICEPS KICKBACK	Begin with 10-sec. squeeze in the extended position, then perform fast reps for 20 sec.	
STANDING ALTERNATING DUMBBELL CURL	Begin with 10-sec. squeeze in the 90-degree position, then perform fast reps for 20 sec.	None
	Repeat this circuit as many times as possible in 7 min.	

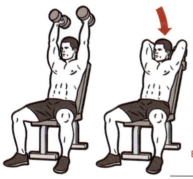

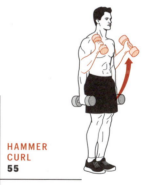

SEATED OVERHEAD DUMBBELL TRICEPS EXTENSION
56

HAMMER CURL
55

58 TRICEPS KICKBACK

54 STANDING ALTERNATING DUMBBELL CURL

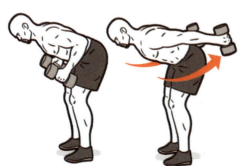

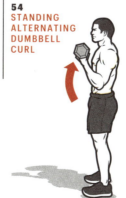

WEIGHTED – ARMS

BIS-AND-TRIS COUNTDOWN BLAST

CIRCUIT 1	WORK	REST
FRENCH PRESS PUSHUP	10 reps	None
DUMBBELL CURL	10 reps	None
Complete 10 rounds of this circuit, decreasing reps by 1 each round. Rest 10 sec. between rounds.		

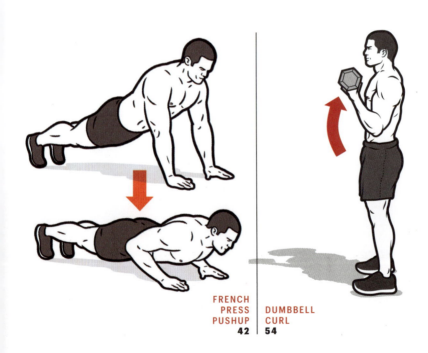

FRENCH
PRESS
PUSHUP
42

DUMBBELL
CURL
54

WEIGHTED – ARMS

ARM TRAINING BASICS

CIRCUIT 1	WORK	REST
DUMBBELL CURL	12 reps	None
SEATED OVERHEAD DUMBBELL TRICEPS EXTENSION	12 reps	None
ZOTTMAN CURL	12 reps (palms up on the way up, palms down on the way down)	None
Complete 4 rounds of this circuit. Rest 30 sec. between rounds.		

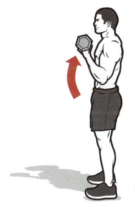
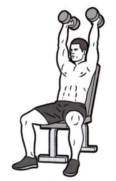

DUMBBELL CURL
54

SEATED OVERHEAD DUMBBELL TRICEPS EXTENSION
56

58
ZOTTMAN CURL

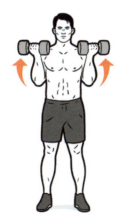
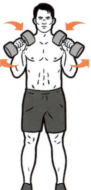
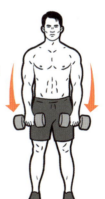

WEIGHTED – ARMS

THE ALL-ANGLES ARM PUMP

CIRCUIT 1	WORK	REST
HAMMER CURL	10 reps	As little as possible
PLANK ALTERNATING ROW-TO-TRICEPS KICKBACK	6 reps	As little as possible
SPEED ALTERNATING DUMBBELL CURL (LIGHT WEIGHTS)	15 reps	As little as possible
CLOSE-GRIP PUSHUP	15 reps	As little as possible
Repeat this circuit as many times as possible in 7 min.		

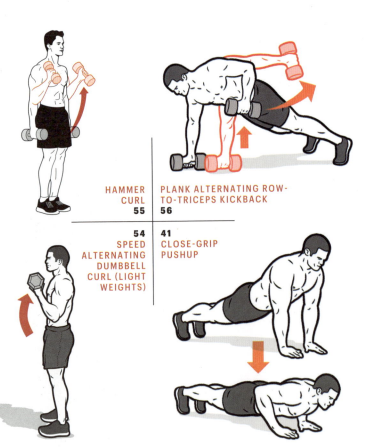

HAMMER CURL
55

PLANK ALTERNATING ROW-TO-TRICEPS KICKBACK
56

54
SPEED ALTERNATING DUMBBELL CURL (LIGHT WEIGHTS)

41
CLOSE-GRIP PUSHUP

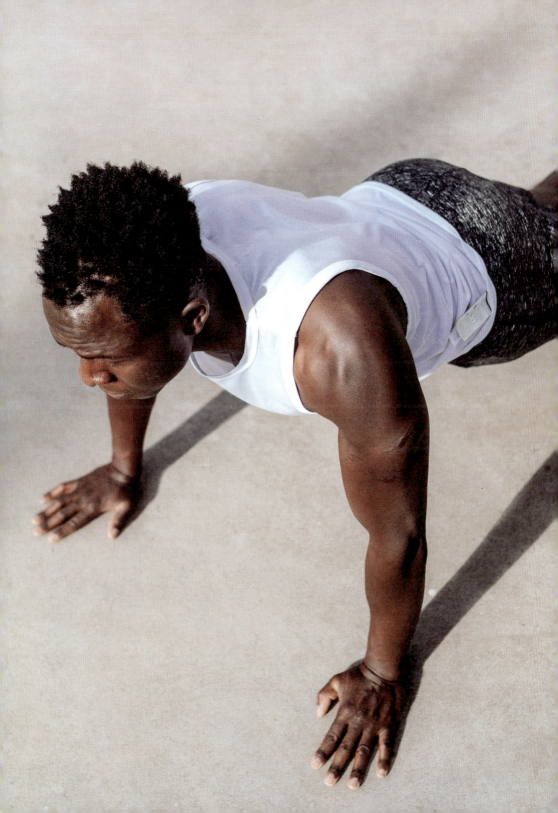

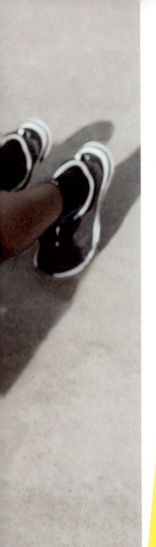

SEVEN-MINUTE
BACK
WORKOUTS

A STRONG, POWERFUL BACK is vital to full-body strength, health, and athleticism. Want to lift something off the floor? Pull yourself over an obstacle? Climb a wall, do a pull-up? Your back muscles are the main movers. For these workouts, you'll be doing a lot of gripping and pulling—two moves that most gym-goers don't get enough of. Move fast between sets—those muscles on the sides of your back (the latissimus dorsi, or lats) and mid-back (the traps and rhomboids, among others) are capable of a lot of work. Make every second count.

BODYWEIGHT – BACK

THE BACK AND REAR-DELTS STABILIZER

EXERCISE	SETS	WORK	REST
SCAPULAR RETRACTION	2	45 sec.	15 sec.
BENT-OVER T	2	45 sec.	15 sec.
3-POINT BEAST	2	45 sec.	15 sec.
BEAR CRAWL	1	45 sec.	15 sec.

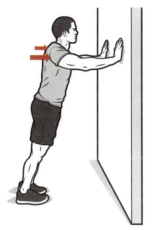

SCAPULAR RETRACTION
44

BENT-OVER T
43

40
3-POINT BEAST

32
BEAR CRAWL

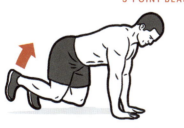

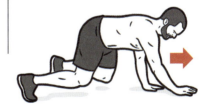

BODYWEIGHT – BACK

ULTIMATE BACK AND CORE MOBILIZER

EXERCISE	SETS	WORK	REST
RAG DOLL	2	45 sec.	15 sec.
BENT-OVER Y	2	45 sec.	15 sec.
BEAR CRAWL	2	45 sec.	15 sec.
BEAST TAP	1	45 sec.	15 sec.

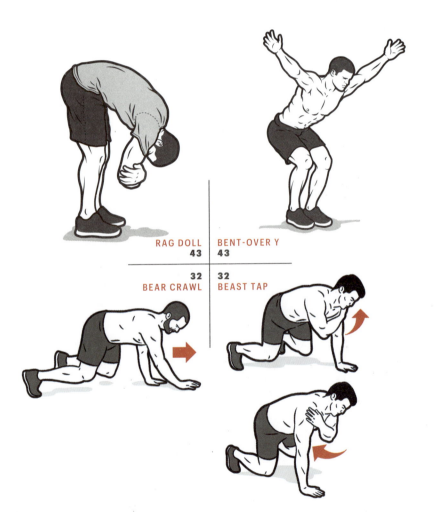

RAG DOLL
43

BENT-OVER Y
43

32
BEAR CRAWL

32
BEAST TAP

BODYWEIGHT – **BACK**

TOTAL POSTERIOR CHAIN CRUSHER

EXERCISE	SETS	WORK	REST
THORACIC ROTATION	1	45 sec. per side	15 sec.
CRAB GRAB	1	45 sec. per side	15 sec.
SIDE PLANK WITH HIP THRUST	1	45 sec. per side	15 sec.
BEAST BOX DRILL	1	45 sec.	15 sec.

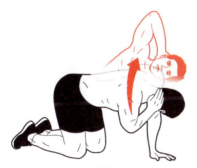

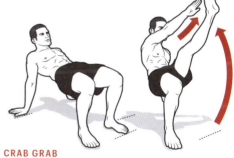

THORACIC ROTATION
68

CRAB GRAB
34

50
SIDE PLANK WITH HIP THRUST

33
BEAST BOX DRILL

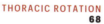

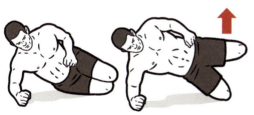

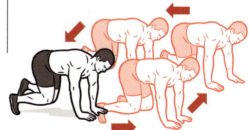

BODYWEIGHT – **BACK**

THE MIDBACK-FOCUSED CIRCUIT

EXERCISE	SETS	WORK	REST
SHOULDER JOINT CIRCLE	2	45 sec.	15 sec.
BENT-OVER W	2	45 sec.	15 sec.
BEAR CRAWL	2	45 sec.	15 sec.
SUPERMAN	2	45 sec.	15 sec.

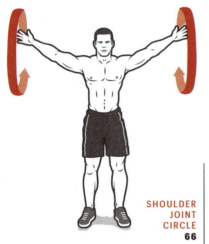

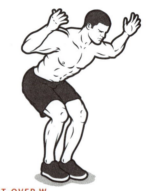

SHOULDER
JOINT
CIRCLE
66

BENT-OVER W
43

32
BEAR CRAWL

44
SUPERMAN

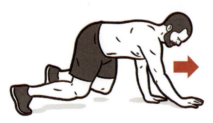

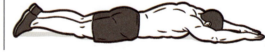

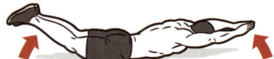

WEIGHTED – **BACK**

THE ROWS AND PRESSES INTERVAL SESSION

CIRCUIT 1	WORK	REST
SINGLE ARM DUMBBELL ROW (R)	40 sec.	20 sec.
SINGLE ARM DUMBBELL ROW (L)	40 sec.	20 sec.
DUMBBELL GLUTE BRIDGE	40 sec.	20 sec.
Complete 2 rounds of this circuit.		

FINISHER	WORK	REST
DUMBBELL SQUAT TO PRESS	60 sec.	None

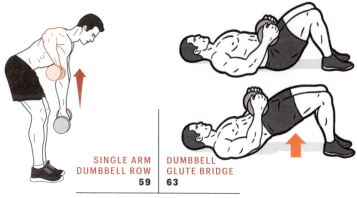

SINGLE ARM
DUMBBELL ROW
59

DUMBBELL
GLUTE BRIDGE
63

63
DUMBBELL SQUAT
TO PRESS

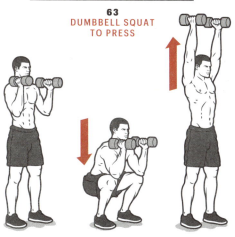

WEIGHTED – **BACK**

BACK AND GLUTES EMOM

CIRCUIT 1	REPS	REST
SINGLE LEG DEADLIFT TO ROW (R)	12–15 reps	This is an EMOM workout. Begin each move at the start of a minute. Complete the reps, then use the remaining time in the minute as your rest.
SINGLE LEG DEADLIFT TO ROW (L)	12–15 reps	
DUMBBELL SWING	20 reps	
Complete 2 rounds of this circuit.		

FINISHER	WORK	REST
DUMBBELL-FACING BURPEE	AMRAP* in 1 min.	None
*As many reps as possible		

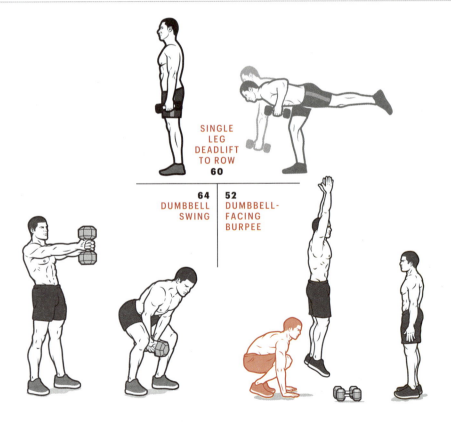

SINGLE LEG DEADLIFT TO ROW
60

64 DUMBBELL SWING

52 DUMBBELL-FACING BURPEE

WEIGHTED – **BACK**

THE TOTAL-BODY BACK BLAST

CIRCUIT 1	WORK	REST
DUMBBELL RENEGADE ROW	30 sec.	15 sec.
TALL KNEELING LATERAL DUMBBELL RAISE	30 sec.	15 sec.
DOUBLE KETTLEBELL SWING	30 sec.	15 sec.
Complete 2 rounds of this circuit.		

FINISHER	WORK	REST
180-DEGREE JUMP	60 sec.	None

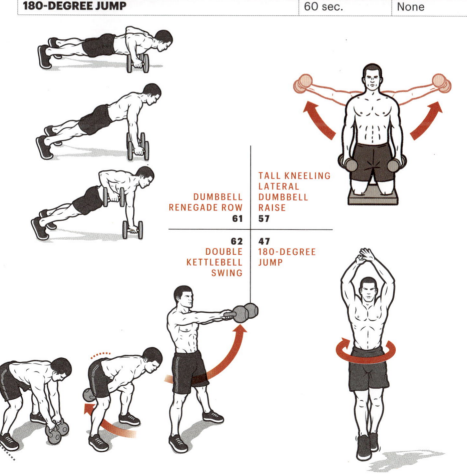

DUMBBELL
RENEGADE ROW
61

TALL KNEELING
LATERAL
DUMBBELL
RAISE
57

62
DOUBLE
KETTLEBELL
SWING

47
180-DEGREE
JUMP

WEIGHTED – BACK

THE FUNCTIONAL BACK ATTACK

CIRCUIT 1	WORK	REST
DEADLIFT TO ROW	30 sec.	15 sec.
HINGE TO DUMBBELL TRICEPS KICKBACK	30 sec.	15 sec.
LUNGE TO FRONT RAISE	30 sec.	15 sec.
Complete 2 rounds of this circuit.		

FINISHER	WORK	REST
DUMBBELL FRONT SQUAT	60 sec.	None

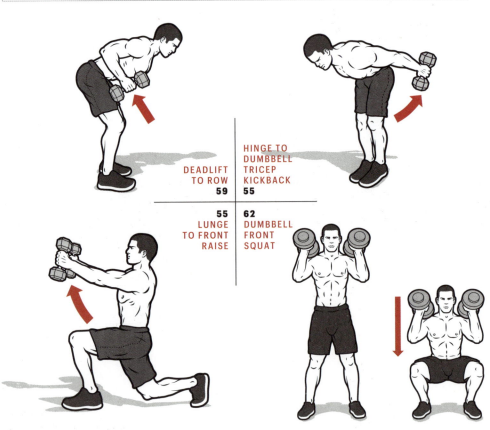

DEADLIFT TO ROW 59

HINGE TO DUMBBELL TRICEP KICKBACK 55

55 LUNGE TO FRONT RAISE

62 DUMBBELL FRONT SQUAT

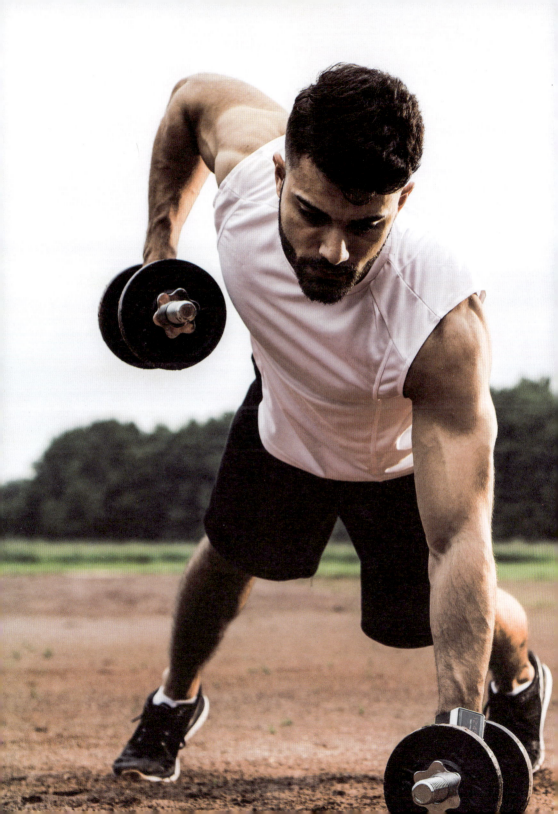

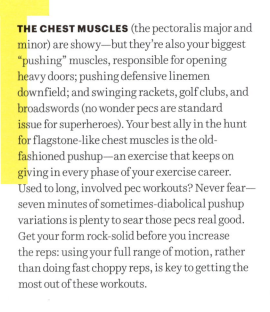

SEVEN-MINUTE
CHEST
WORKOUTS

THE CHEST MUSCLES (the pectoralis major and minor) are showy—but they're also your biggest "pushing" muscles, responsible for opening heavy doors; pushing defensive linemen downfield; and swinging rackets, golf clubs, and broadswords (no wonder pecs are standard issue for superheroes). Your best ally in the hunt for flagstone-like chest muscles is the old-fashioned pushup—an exercise that keeps on giving in every phase of your exercise career. Used to long, involved pec workouts? Never fear—seven minutes of sometimes-diabolical pushup variations is plenty to sear those pecs real good. Get your form rock-solid before you increase the reps: using your full range of motion, rather than doing fast choppy reps, is key to getting the most out of these workouts.

BODYWEIGHT – CHEST

THE PUSHUP MECHANICAL DROPSET EMOM

7-MIN. EMOM	WORK	REST
PLYO PUSHUP	4 reps	This is an EMOM workout. Begin each move at the start of a minute. Complete the reps, then use the remaining time in the minute as your rest.
PUSHUP	6 reps	
DEADSTOP PUSHUP	8 reps	

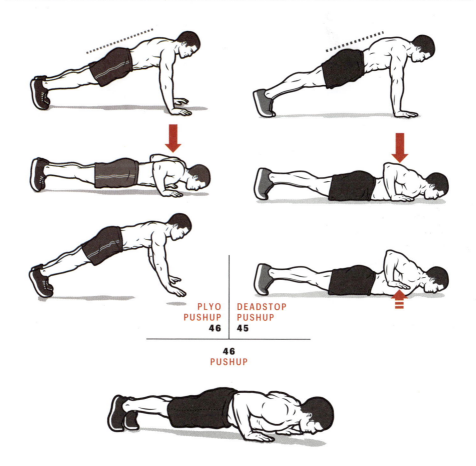

PLYO PUSHUP 46   DEADSTOP PUSHUP 45

46 PUSHUP

BODYWEIGHT – CHEST

PUSHUP-AND-BURPEE HELL

CIRCUIT 1	WORK	REST
PUSHUP	30 sec.	30 sec.
BURPEE	30 sec.	30 sec.

Complete 5 rounds of this circuit, decreasing pushup reps each round as follows:

Round 2	15 Pushups
Round 3	10 Pushups
Round 4	10 Pushups
Round 5	5 Pushups

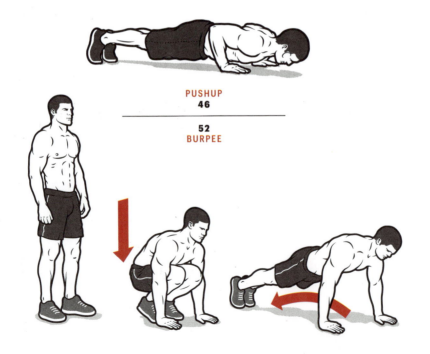

PUSHUP
46

52
BURPEE

BODYWEIGHT – CHEST

THE QUICK-INTERVAL PUSHUP CRUSHER

7-MIN. ETOT	WORK	REST
T-STOP PUSHUP	4 reps	This is an ETOT (every time on the time) workout. Begin each move at the start of a 30-sec. timer. Complete the reps, then use the remaining time as your rest.
PLYO PUSHUP	4 reps	

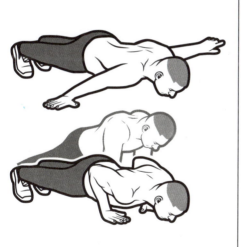

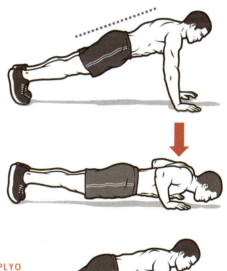

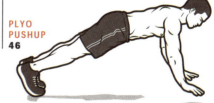

T-STOP   PLYO
PUSHUP   PUSHUP
46   **46**

BODYWEIGHT – CHEST

DEATH BY PUSHUP INTERVALS

CIRCUIT 1	WORK	REST
DEADSTOP PUSHUP	30 sec.	None
T-STOP PUSHUP	30 sec.	None
PUSHUP	30 sec.	None
Complete 3 rounds of this circuit. Rest 60 sec. between rounds.		

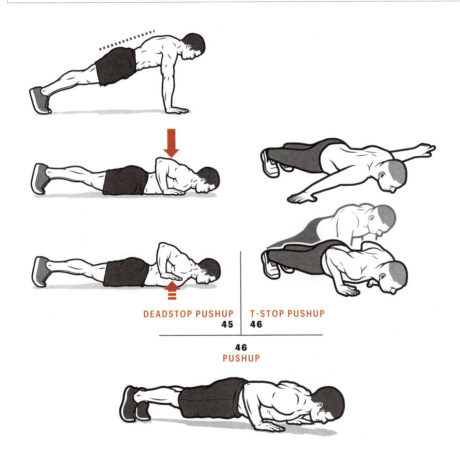

DEADSTOP PUSHUP
45

T-STOP PUSHUP
46

46
PUSHUP

WEIGHTED – CHEST

THE DUMBBELLS-AND-PUSHUPS CHEST CRUSHER

CIRCUIT 1	WORK	REST
FLOOR PRESS	40 sec.	None
DEADSTOP PUSHUP	30 sec.	None
PLYO PUSHUP	20 sec.	None
Complete 3 rounds of this circuit. Rest 60 sec. between rounds.		

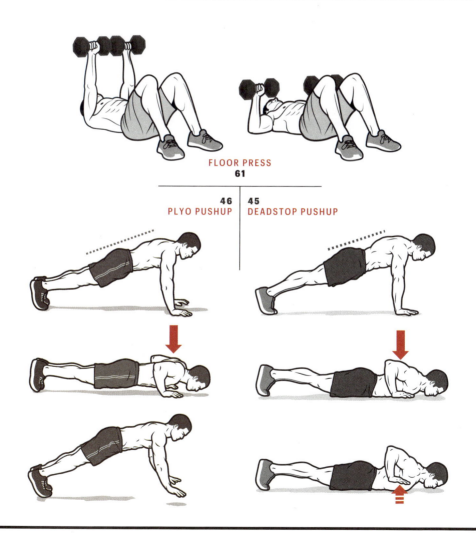

FLOOR PRESS
61

46
PLYO PUSHUP

45
DEADSTOP PUSHUP

WEIGHTED – CHEST

THE PRESS-FOCUSED UPPER-BODY PUMP

LADDER	WORK	REST
FLOOR PRESS	10 reps	None
CLOSE-GRIP FLOOR PRESS	10 reps	None
RENEGADE ROW	10 reps	None
Complete 10 rounds of this circuit, decreasing reps by 1 each round.		

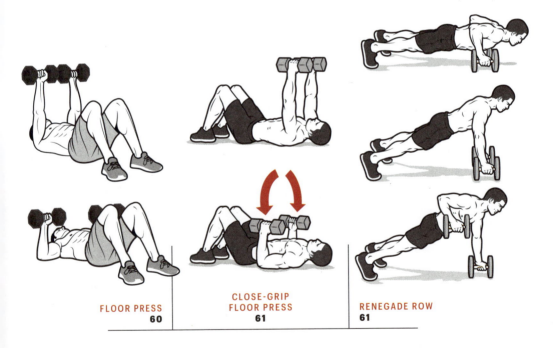

FLOOR PRESS
60

CLOSE-GRIP
FLOOR PRESS
61

RENEGADE ROW
61

WEIGHTED – CHEST

THE TABATA PRESS SESSION

CIRCUIT 1	WORK	REST
CLOSE-GRIP FLOOR PRESS	20 sec.	10 sec.
DEADSTOP PUSHUP	20 sec.	10 sec.
PLYO PUSHUP	20 sec.	10 sec.
Complete 4 rounds of this circuit.		

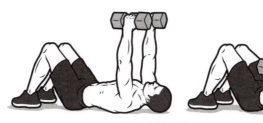

CLOSE-GRIP FLOOR PRESS
60

45
DEADSTOP PUSHUP

46
PLYO PUSHUP

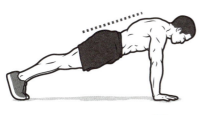

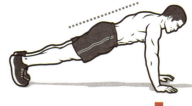

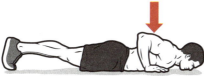

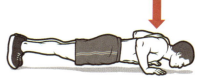

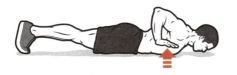

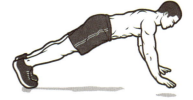

WEIGHTED – CHEST

THE TERRIBLE 10S CHEST EMOM

7-MIN. EMOM	REPS	REST
FLOOR PRESS	10 reps	This is an EMOM workout. Begin each move at the start of a minute. Complete the reps, then use the remaining time in the minute as your rest.
DEADSTOP PUSHUP	10 reps	
PUSHUP	10 reps	
FLOOR PRESS	10 reps	
DEADSTOP PUSHUP	10 reps	
PUSHUP	10 reps	
BURPEE	AMRAP for 60 sec.	

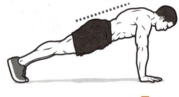

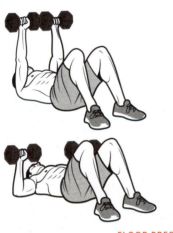

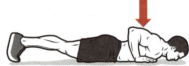

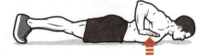

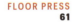

FLOOR PRESS
61

DEADSTOP PUSHUP
45

46
PUSHUP

52
BURPEE

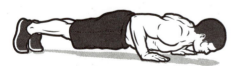

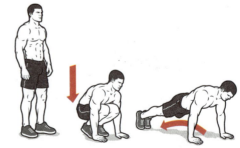

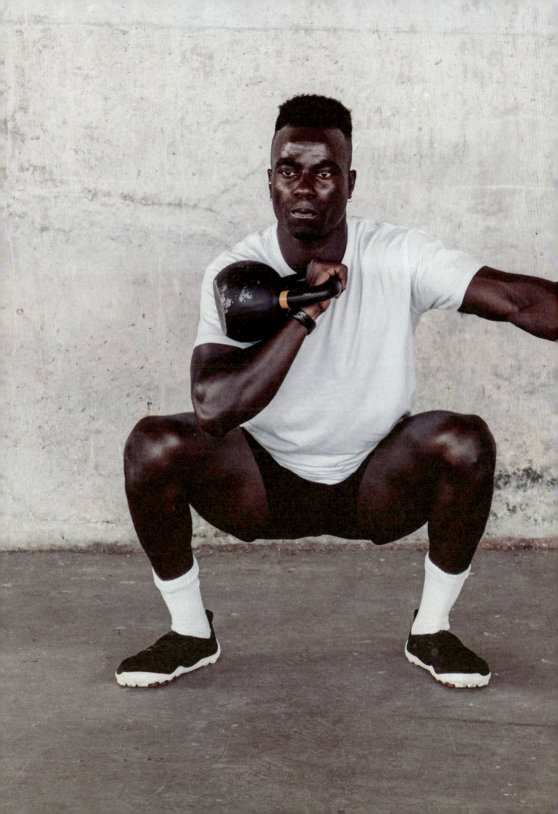

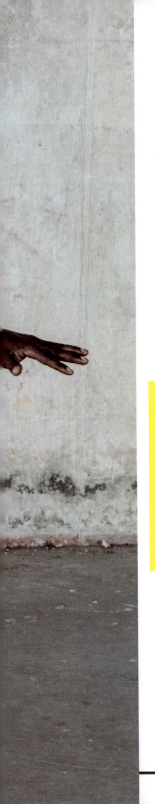

SEVEN-MINUTE
LEG
WORKOUTS

FOR HEAVEN'S SAKE, don't skip leg day—especially if it only lasts seven minutes. Something on the order of 60 percent of your muscle tissue resides below your waist, so if you're serious about staying strong, lean, and athletic, make these workouts a priority. Many people turn to leg machines and isolation moves to build muscular legs, but the best way to build strong wheels is with your feet solidly on the ground, with variations on squats, lunges, hip thrusts, and deadlifts. Your quads (front thighs), hamstrings (rear thighs), glutes (butt muscles), and calves are all thick, dense muscles, capable of carrying your entire bodyweight around for long periods. For best results, you need to steel yourself for a little discomfort—okay, pain—to make those muscles strengthen and grow further. Upside: It's just seven minutes.

BODYWEIGHT – LEGS

THE STRENGTH AND POWER CHIPPER

CIRCUIT 1	WORK	REST
SHIN BOX TO TALL KNEELING (R)	5 reps	None
SHIN BOX TO TALL KNEELING (L)	5 reps	None
ALTERNATING REVERSE LUNGE	30 reps	None
JUMP SQUAT	25 reps	None
BROAD JUMP	12 reps	None
Complete 2 rounds of this circuit.		

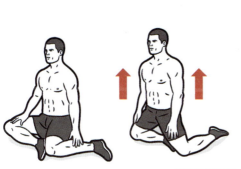

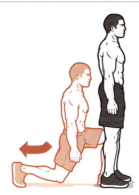

SHIN BOX TO
TALL KNEELING
49

ALTERNATING
REVERSE LUNGE
49

49
JUMP
SQUAT

52
BROAD
JUMP

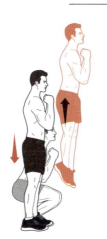

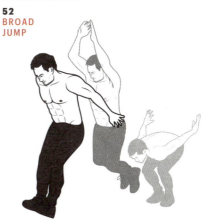

BODYWEIGHT – LEGS

MULTIPLANAR LEG INTERVALS

CIRCUIT 1	WORK	REST
TOE TOUCH	30 sec.	None
HIP HINGE	30 sec.	None
CALF RAISE	30 sec.	None
Complete 2 rounds of this circuit.		

4-MIN. EMOM	WORK	REST
LATERAL LUNGE	10 reps per side	This is an EMOM series. Begin a set of lateral lunges at the start of a minute. Complete the reps, then use the remaining time in the minute as your rest.

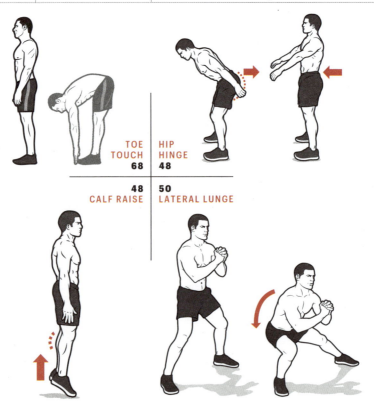

TOE TOUCH **68**

HIP HINGE **48**

48 CALF RAISE

50 LATERAL LUNGE

BODYWEIGHT – LEGS

LOWER-BODY MOBILITY, STRENGTH, AND POWER

EXERCISE	SETS	WORK	REST
INCHWORM TO RUNNER'S STRETCH	1	60 sec.	None
BODYWEIGHT SQUAT	1	60 sec.	None
SKATER LUNGE	1	60 sec.	None
Complete 2 rounds of this circuit. Rest 60 sec. between rounds.			

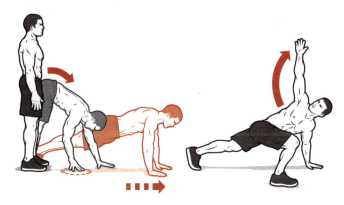

INCHWORM TO RUNNER'S STRETCH
48

47
BODYWEIGHT SQUAT

50
SKATER LUNGE

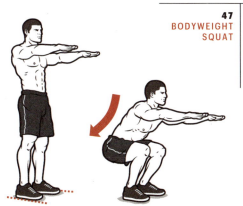

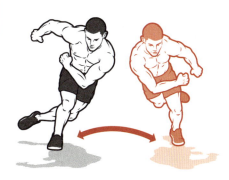

BODYWEIGHT – LEGS

LOWER-BODY CONTROL AND POWER

CIRCUIT 1	WORK	REST
SIDE PLANK WITH HIP THRUST	30 sec.	None
SPLIT SQUAT ISO HOLD (R)	30 sec.	None
SPLIT SQUAT ISO HOLD (L)	30 sec.	None
Complete 2 rounds of this circuit.		

SUPERSET 1	WORK	REST
180-DEGREE JUMP	30 sec.	None
ALTERNATING LUNGE	30 sec.	None
Complete 3 rounds of this superset.		

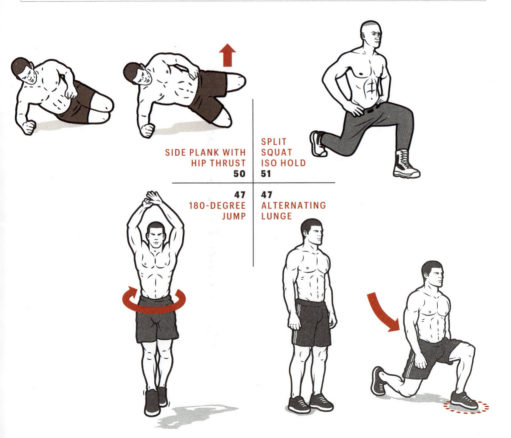

SIDE PLANK WITH
HIP THRUST
50

SPLIT
SQUAT
ISO HOLD
51

47
180-DEGREE
JUMP

47
ALTERNATING
LUNGE

WEIGHTED – LEGS

THE QUAD-HAMSTRING CRUSHER CIRCUIT

CIRCUIT 1	WORK	REST
DUMBBELL FRONT SQUAT	8 reps	None
DUMBBELL SWING	16 reps	None
Complete 4 rounds of this circuit.		

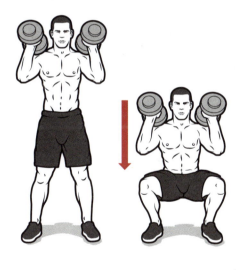

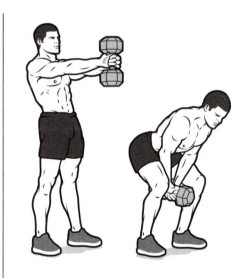

DUMBBELL
FRONT SQUAT
62

DUMBBELL
SWING
64

WEIGHTED – **LEGS**

THE HIGH-REP LEG AMRAP

CIRCUIT 1	WORK	REST
GOBLET ALTERNATING REVERSE LUNGE	20 reps	None
SUMO SQUAT STRETCH	60 sec.	None
Repeat this circuit as many times as possible in 7 min.		

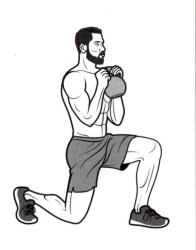

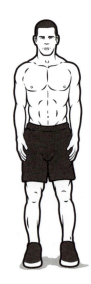

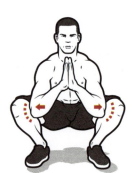

GOBLET
ALTERNATING
REVERSE LUNGE
64

SUMO
SQUAT
STRETCH
51

WEIGHTED – **LEGS**

SINGLE-LEG STRENGTH AND ATHLETICISM

CIRCUIT 1	WORK	REST
SINGLE LEG ROMANIAN DEADLIFT (R)	8 reps	30 sec.
SINGLE LEG ROMANIAN DEADLIFT (L)	8 reps	30 sec.
DUMBBELL JUMP SQUAT	16 reps	30 sec.
Complete 3 rounds of this circuit.		

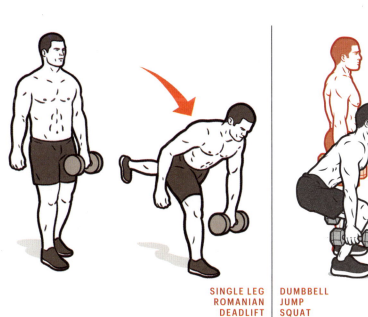

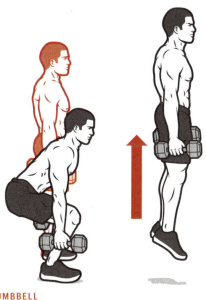

SINGLE LEG
ROMANIAN
DEADLIFT
64

DUMBBELL
JUMP
SQUAT
62

WEIGHTED – **LEGS**

DOUBLE-KETTLEBELL LEG MADNESS

CIRCUIT 1	WORK	REST
DOUBLE RACK SQUAT	25 reps	None
DOUBLE KETTLEBELL SWING	25 reps	None
Complete 2 rounds of this circuit. Rest 2 min. between rounds.		

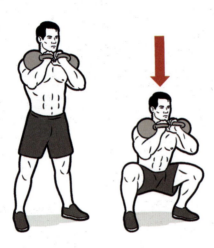

DOUBLE RACK SQUAT
62

62
DOUBLE KETTLEBELL SWING

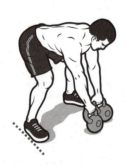 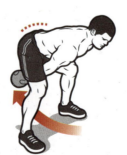 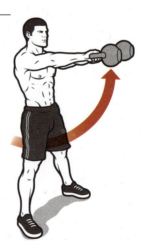

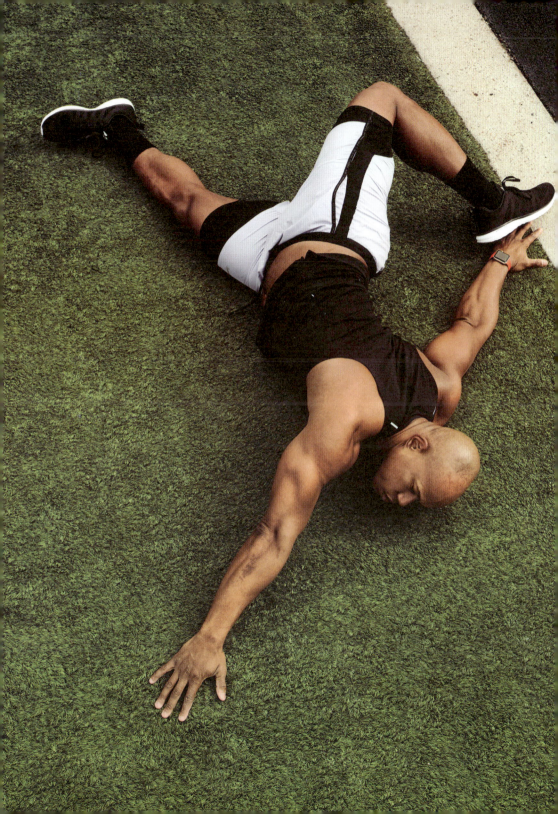

SEVEN-MINUTE
RECOVERY
WORKOUTS

HARD WORKOUTS ARE a form of stress: When you lift, you break down muscle tissue, which your body rebuilds—plus a little extra—in the hours and days that follow. Recovery workouts have the opposite effect: Instead of breaking down muscle tissue, you're bathing it in oxygenated blood, flushing out metabolites, reducing muscle soreness, and speeding recovery at the same time. You don't need a lot of time to do that—active recovery sessions that are too long can be counterproductive. Do these workouts anytime, anywhere—even piecemeal, in one- or two-minute sessions. Consider them "secret sauce" workouts— force multipliers that amplify the results of your strength- and muscle-building workouts.

RECOVERY

TOTAL-BODY MOBILITY AND STABILITY

EXERCISE	SETS	WORK	REST
SUPINE LEG SWITCH	1	45 sec. per side	15 sec.
PRONE SHOULDER IR/ER	1	45 sec. per side	15 sec.
COBRA STRETCH	2	45 sec.	15 sec.
LUNGE STRETCH	1	45 sec. per side	15 sec.

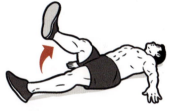

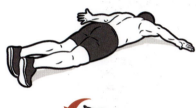

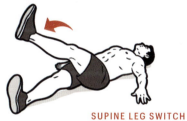

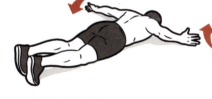

SUPINE LEG SWITCH
69

PRONE SHOULDER IR/ER
67

67
COBRA STRETCH

67
LUNGE STRETCH

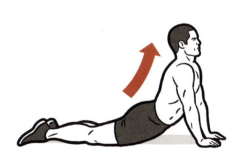

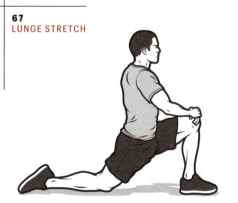

RECOVERY

THE LOWER-BODY MOVE-AND-GROOVE

EXERCISE	SETS	WORK	REST
HIP HINGE	1	45 sec.	15 sec.
KNEE JOINT CIRCLE	1	45 sec.	15 sec.
INCHWORM TO RUNNER'S STRETCH	2	45 sec. per side	15 sec.
LATERAL LUNGE	1	45 sec. per side	15 sec.

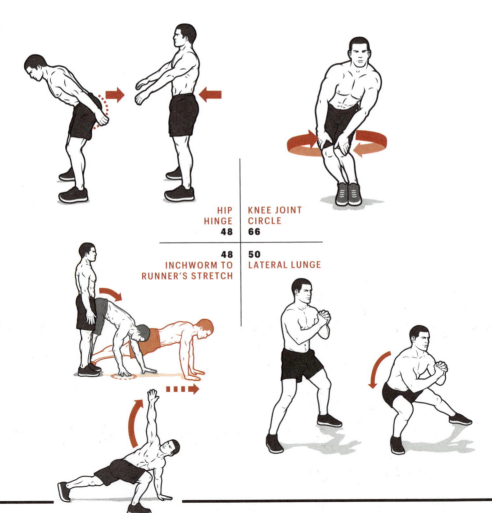

HIP HINGE
48

KNEE JOINT CIRCLE
66

48
INCHWORM TO RUNNER'S STRETCH

50
LATERAL LUNGE

RECOVERY

THE ULTIMATE HIP-RELAXING FLEX

EXERCISE	SETS	WORK	REST
TOE TOUCH	2	45 sec.	15 sec.
REVERSE LUNGE	1	45 sec. per side	15 sec.
WORLD'S GREATEST STRETCH	1	45 sec. per side	15 sec.
3-LEGGED DOG	1	45 sec. per side	15 sec.

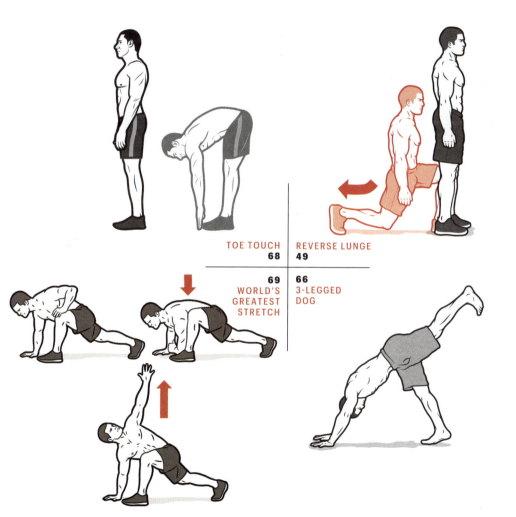

TOE TOUCH
68

REVERSE LUNGE
49

69
WORLD'S
GREATEST
STRETCH

66
3-LEGGED
DOG

RECOVERY

FULL-BODY MOBILITY

EXERCISE	SETS	WORK	REST
HIP JOINT CIRCLE	1	45 sec.	15 sec.
INCHWORM TO RUNNER'S STRETCH	1	45 sec. per side	15 sec.
SHIN BOX TO TALL KNEELING	1	45 sec. per side	15 sec.
SIDE-LYING T-SPINE ROTATION	1	45 sec. per side	15 sec.

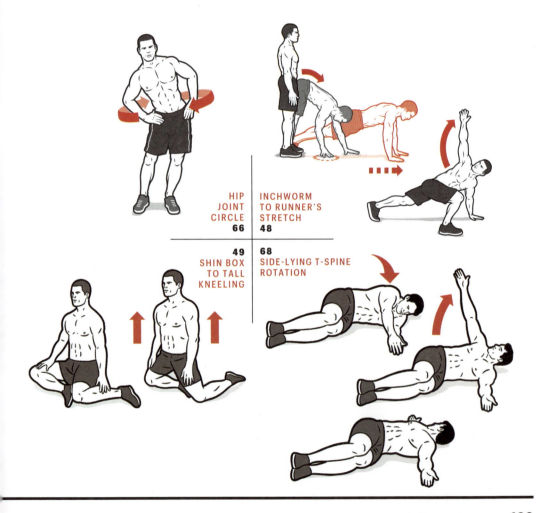

HIP JOINT CIRCLE
66

INCHWORM TO RUNNER'S STRETCH
48

49
SHIN BOX TO TALL KNEELING

68
SIDE-LYING T-SPINE ROTATION

WORKOUT LOG

DATE _____

WORKOUT _____
_____

DATE _____

WORKOUT _____
_____

DATE _____

WORKOUT _____
_____

DATE _____

WORKOUT _____
_____

DATE _____

WORKOUT _____
_____

DATE _____

WORKOUT _____
_____

DATE _____

WORKOUT _____
_____

DATE _____

WORKOUT _____
_____

DATE _____

WORKOUT _____
_____

DATE _____

WORKOUT _____
_____

DATE _____

WORKOUT _____
_____

DATE _____

WORKOUT _____
_____

DATE _____

WORKOUT _____
_____

DATE _____

WORKOUT _____
_____

DATE _____

WORKOUT _____
_____

DATE _____

WORKOUT _____
_____

DATE _____

WORKOUT _____
_____

DATE _____

WORKOUT _____
_____

DATE _____

WORKOUT _____
_____

DATE _____

WORKOUT _____
_____

DATE _____

WORKOUT _____
_____

DATE _____

WORKOUT _____
_____

DATE _____

WORKOUT _____
_____

DATE _____

WORKOUT _____
_____

DATE _____

WORKOUT _____
_____

DATE _____

WORKOUT _____
_____

DATE _____

WORKOUT _____
_____

DATE _____

WORKOUT _____
_____

© 2022 by Hearst Magazines, Inc.

Men's Health is a registered trademark of
Hearst Magazines, Inc.

Book design by Gillian MacLeod

Library of Congress Cataloging-in-Publication Data
is on file with the publisher.

ISBN 978-1-955710-10-7

Printed in China

2 4 6 8 10 9 7 5 3 1 hardcover

HEARST

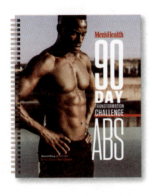 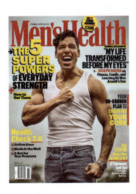 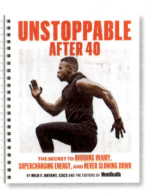